OXFORD MEDICAL PUBLICATIONS

IMMUNOLOGY SIMPLIFIED

GW00724806

Immunology Simplified

T. R. BOWRY
MB, MRCPath

Senior Lecturer
WHO Immunology Research & Training Centre
Department of Pathology, University of Nairobi

OXFORD
OXFORD UNIVERSITY PRESS
IBADAN DELHI

Oxford University Press, Walton Street, Oxford OX2 6DP

OXFORD LONDON GLASGOW
NEW YORK TORONTO MELBOURNE WELLINGTON
IBADAN NAIROBI DAR ES SALAAM LUSAKA CAPE TOWN
KUALA LUMPUR SINGAPORE JAKARTA HONG KONG TOKYO
DELHI BOMBAY CALCUTTA MADRAS KARACHI

ISBN 0 19 261148 8

Published outside of East Africa
by Oxford University Press, by arrangement
with the African Medical and Research Foundation
P.O. Box 30125, Nairobi, Kenya
1977
Reprinted 1979

Printed in Great Britain
by J. W. Arrowsmith Ltd., Bristol

FOREWORD

Historically the science of immunology originated in experience that persons who recovered from epidemic diseases were resistant—'immune'—to further attacks of the same diseases; this experience initiated empirical trials to protect people against such diseases. Only when micro-organisms were recognized as agents responsible for infectious diseases, however, was a more scientific basis available for studies of acquired resistance to infections and the development of different types of vaccines.

The two main effectors of protection—antibodies and cellular components—were already known at the end of last century. More detailed studies performed in this century clarified the properties of the foreign (non-self) substances—'antigens'—which initiate immune responses, the structure of antibodies and their binding with antigens into antigen-antibody complexes, the interactions of these with other humoral factors (complement) as well as the cellular components involved, and their ultrastructure and the receptors on their surfaces. It is only recently, however, that the mechanisms of how the immune system operates and how it is regulated and controlled have come to be better understood, and I believe that much still remains to be learnt.

The immune response of the organism is its principal physiological adaptive mechanism of host defence against non-self substances, in other words its main function is guarding and monitoring the identity of the body; unfortunately, under certain circumstances, it can also induce pathophysiological—better termed immunopathological—reactions causing harm to the host. The immunological reactivity of the organism is also very important in transplantation, and methods of suppressing and perhaps preventing possible undesirable reactions have been intensively studied. There is even hope that further studies of the immune system may help in the fight against cancer.

This brief reference to the different situations in which immune responses are involved shows the complexity and the broadening scope of immunology, how it has developed from attempts to *increase* immune responses (e.g. with vaccines, some of which have proved very effective) in order to protect the host against infections, *via* efforts to *control* the diseases of the immune system (allergies, autoimmunity, immuno-deficiencies), to attempts to *suppress* undesirable immune responses (prevention of transplant rejection). It is to be hoped that the most recent findings will facilitate manipulation of immune responses according to the need of the organism.

Dr Tula Bowry, my former student and present colleague, has prepared this short survey of Immunology for those who want to understand the constituents and mechanisms of the immunological reactivity of the organism and their applications to the practical clinical problems which we face. I would like to congratulate her on having managed to describe this complicated system in such a short, intelligible, and 'simplified' form, without omitting any important part of the latest knowledge on the subject.

Department of Pathology
University of Nairobi

Professor V. Houba, MD, DSc
Head, WHO Immunology
Research and Training Centre

PREFACE

Two difficulties face the student of any rapidly developing subject. Firstly the advancing edge tends to be alarmingly complicated, and secondly it takes time for new concepts to be accepted and take their place in easily comprehensible form among the basic essentials of the subject. There is thus an ever-present danger of the whole subject being regarded as 'difficult' from the start, an attitude which prevents it ever being enjoyable.

Immunology is without doubt the subject of the future. There is almost no field of biological research, except the most mechanical, which is not forced to use immunological principles in order to make progress. Not to feel at ease with immunological concepts these days is to be handicapped right from the outset.

In this book, which is based on several years' experience of teaching both undergraduates and postgraduates, my aim has been to set out the fundamentals of immunology without frightening the reader, and at the same time to explain the way they apply today to the fields of human and veterinary medicine, and general biology.

Immunology is changing almost daily. If the reader gains from this book sufficient familiarity with the part it plays in clinical allergy, immunity to infections, transplant work, and cancer research to be encouraged to keep up with further advances as they are reported, I shall have succeeded in what I set out to do.

Nairobi   Tula Bowry

ACKNOWLEDGMENTS

This book would never have seen the light of day had the short series of articles in *Medicine Digest* two years ago not been so kindly received, and had I not been encouraged to expand and revise them into the present volume by my colleagues, especially by Professor V. Houba, to whom I am also indebted for the foreword.

Both the original articles and the book owe their form to the patient and persistent editorial help of Dr Hugh de Glanville and the infinite pains taken by Miss N. Dames over the diagrams and the figures.

I wish to thank all my past students, for it is from the pleasurable experience of teaching them that the book has taken shape. Finally I must thank *Medicine Digest* for waiving their copyright and the African Medical & Research Foundation for underwriting the publication.

T.R.B.

TABLE OF CONTENTS

Chapter one

BIOLOGICAL ASPECTS OF IMMUNITY

Introduction

Immunology is the study of the processes by which the body, surrounded as it is by a polluted external environment, defends and maintains the constancy of its internal milieu against invasion by 'foreign' organisms, or the mutation or development of unwanted cells or cell products within itself.

While part of immunology concerns the search for vaccines for the vast range of infectious microbial and parasitic disease, the subject is expanding in the understanding of the pathogenesis, diagnosis, and treatment of hypersensitivity states, connective tissue diseases, autoimmune diseases, immunodeficiency states, and cancer. Finally, advances in immunology have made possible the transplantation of healthy organs to replace diseased ones, a field in which the search for further improvement continues.

Particular advances have been made in the last two decades, with the definition of the functions of the lymphocytes—T cells dominating cell-mediated

immunity, B cells responsible for humoral immunity—
and of the co-operation between these two forms,
and that between macrophages and lymphocytes.
This chapter deals with these discoveries.

What began as an attempt to potentiate the body's
defences against infectious diseases by vaccination has
developed into study of the whole functioning of the
immune system, in order on the one hand to enhance
immune responses against infection or against cancer,
on the other hand to suppress unwanted immune
responses in hypersensitivity states or to allow transplantations.

Immunity (*Fig 1.1*)

'Immunity' is a term which originally implied exemp-
tion from military service or taxes; it was introduced
into medicine to refer to those people who did not
get further attacks of smallpox or plague once they
had had the disease. In a wider sense the term refers
to the resistance of a host organism to invasive pathogens or their toxic products.

Immunity is divided into two main types:

● non-specific immunity (sometimes called 'innate immunity') which includes the general common protective reactions
of the organism against invasion, and

● specific immunity.

Invertebrates have only non-specific immunity,
while vertebrates show both types, and indeed the
two are closely linked functionally in mammals and
man.

Non-specific immunity

Non-specific immunity does not involve specific recog-

Fig 1.1

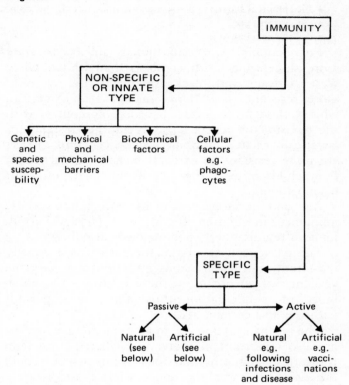

nition of the foreign agent. The methods by which it operates include (*Fig 1.1*):

• species or genetic insusceptibility to certain pathogens (e.g. man does not catch fowlpox, dogs cannot be given measles);

● physical barriers to infection—skin, mucous membranes;
● biochemical barriers—lysozymes, stomach acid, the complement system, etc;
● cellular mechanisms.

For example, American Indians and Negroes are more susceptible to tuberculosis than whites, while West Africans and black Americans are relatively more resistant to *P vivax* malaria than American whites, though the former have had no contact with the parasite for generations. As another instance of genetically related immunity, sickle cell trait carriers are more resistant to cerebral malaria, in particular, than children with the full complement of adult haemoglobin.

Age and hormonal status also affect non-specific immunity; in children, for instance, laryngeal papillomas often disappear spontaneously at puberty.

The pathogenicity of the foreign agent is equally important, and spontaneous mutation may vary the virulence of an organism; there is always the possibility of a non-pathogen becoming an important pathogen in a community.

The mechanical skin and mucous membrane barriers are also important in protection: ciliated epithelium traps dust and other noxious agents which would otherwise reach the lungs and possibly cause disease.

The biochemically active antimicrobial mechanisms in the blood, tissue fluids, intestinal secretions, sweat, and tears include interferon, hydrochloric acid, lysozymes, basic polypeptides, and the complement-properdin system.

The phagocytes—the polymorph neutrophils and mononuclear macrophages—play an important part in

the body's non-specific immune mechanisms in vertebrates.

Specific immunity (*Fig 1.1*)

This, as has long been taught, is divided into passive
and active immunity, both of which may be either
natural or artificial.

Passive immunity involves either the transfer of
antibody or, in some diseases, of sensitized cells from
an immune to a non-immune person. Natural passive
immunity is transferred from mother to child across
the placenta or in the colostrum. Artificially it is
transferred therapeutically by various antitoxins or
gammaglobulins, as in the treatment of tetanus,
diphtheria, gas gangrene, snake bite, and immunodeficient states. In certain diseases the passive transfer
of immunity by antibody is not successful—tuberculosis is an example—and immunity can only be transferred, as just mentioned, by white cells from an
immune person.

In either case, passive immunity is of short dur-
ation, depending on the life span in the recipient of
the antibody or cells transferred. Once it disappears,
the host is again susceptible to the disease.

Active immunity

The three essential characteristics of active immunity
are:

- recognition
- specificity
- memory.

Recognition

Recognition of foreign agents and substances as distinct from self tissues and proteins is an important characteristic differentiating non-specific from adaptive immunity. The substances recognized are termed 'antigens' which are defined as substances which stimulate an immune response and react specifically with the resultant antibodies or cells. Some low molecular weight substances known as *haptens*, however, are unable by themselves to stimulate a primary response on introduction into the body unless they are conjugated with a larger 'carrier' molecule. Once this initial response has been stimulated, however, the hapten alone is capable of reacting with the resultant antibody and sensitized cells.

Immunogenicity, or the capacity of an antigen (or hapten + carrier) to stimulate an immune response, is determined by such factors as molecular size, chemical constitution, optical configuration, and the spatial folding of its surface. The immunogenicity is also affected by the site of entry to the body, and the rate of breakdown of the agent in the body.

Proteins are potent immunogens, carbohydrates weak, and lipids completely non-immunogenic, unless linked with protein or carbohydrate or both.

The cells in the body which recognize antigens are the small lymphocytes, therefore called 'immunocompetent' cells. These are actively motile but not phagocytic, and have no well developed endoplasmic reticulum, unlike, as we shall see later, plasma cells. They form 35–40% of the circulating white blood cells, but a much larger pool exists in the lymphoid tissues. Some lymphocytes have a life span measured in years, unlike red cells (see also later).

Functionally there are at least two main subtypes of lymphocytes in the body called the 'T' lymphocytes for *Thymus-derived lymphocytes*, and the 'B' lymphocytes for the *Bone marrow-derived lymphocytes*, which are derived from a common haemopoietic stem cell (*Fig 1.2*).

T lymphocytes

Lymphocytes are derived from haemopoietic stem cells, which originate in the yolk sac of the ovum and the liver of the embryo, whence they migrate to bone marrow, which is then the only source of stem cells in the fetus, newborn, child, and adult. At about the time of birth (earlier in man, later in some animals) a population of lymphoid stem cells derived from the haemopoietic stem cells migrates from the bone marrow to the thymus, where it multiplies extensively, producing cells which differentiate into immunocompetent T cells—Thymus-derived small lymphocytes. These T cells leave the thymus to circulate permanently in the blood and in the peripheral lymphoid organs. T cells are, as we said in the introduction, primarily responsible for cell-mediated immunity.

This process of cellular migration to the thymus and thymic processing starts in human beings in fetal life, is fairly active in early childhood, but proceeds slowly thereafter. In animals such as mice, however, the seeding of immunocompetent T cells from thymus to secondary lymph organs does not begin until after birth, which provides us with a useful model for cellular manipulations; thymectomy in the mouse at birth results in a permanent deficiency of

T lymphocytes and impaired ability to develop cell-mediated immunity and to reject grafts.

The neonatally thymectomized mouse also has a reduced capacity for humoral antibody response because, although it has a normal complement of B lymphocytes (see below), these require co-operating helper T cells to function properly. Its ability to resist infection in general is therefore also impaired, and such animals become stunted and wasted unless reared in a germ-free environment.

This immunological deficit can be partly, but not completely, remedied by giving cell-free thymic extracts; this suggests that hormones from the thymus may play some part in the differentiation of T cells.

B lymphocytes

Another population of lymphoid stem cells arising from the haemopoietic stem cells in bone marrow undergoes a process of proliferation and differentiation at a site as yet unknown in mammals but known to be the *Bursa of Fabricius* (located in the hindgut) in birds. There is some evidence from rodents that in mammals this cell line may in fact proliferate and differentiate in, as well as arise from, bone marrow, and these cells are known as B cells—Bursa or Bone marrow-derived small lymphocytes. When B lymphocytes are stimulated by an antigen, blast transformation and then proliferation of the cells occurs resulting in memory cells, which resemble and are indistinguishable from small lymphocytes, and plasma cells. Plasma cells synthesize and secrete antibodies throughout their short life span of 18–48 hours. Thus, B cells are responsible for humoral (non-cellular) antibody-mediated immunity. To respond to most biologi-

Fig 1.2 Derivation of T and B lymphocytes
(Modified from Essential Immunology by I. Roitt, 2nd edn, Blackwell, courtesy author and publishers.)

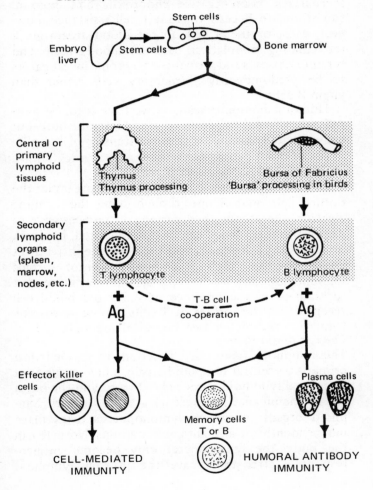

cal antigens, B cells require T cell co-operation. A few antigenic substances, such as pneumococcal poly-saccharides, gram-negative endotoxin, and dextran, can stimulate B cells without T cell assistance, however. Most of the B cells in the blood-stream are a recirculating population between blood-stream and lymphoid tissues and are believed by some investigators to be predominantly B memory cells rather than virgin B cells.

Humoral immunity can, as we have seen, be passively transferred in serum to a non-immune host, but cell-mediated immunity requires transfer of lymphocytes, or of an extract from them.

Distinction between T and B cells

T and B lymphocytes cannot be told apart under the normal light microscope, though under the scanning electron microscope their surface differences serve to distinguish them. They can be differentiated, however, in other ways depending on their surface differences and properties, such as demonstration of surface immunoglobulins on B cells by immunofluorescent techniques, or the presence of sheep red blood cell receptors on the surface of T cells, shown by rosette-formation techniques (see Technical appendix).

The lymphoid tissues

The lymphoid tissues are functionally divided into primary or central lymphoid tissue, and secondary or peripheral lymphoid tissue. The thymus and the bursa (or its mammalian equivalent) are the primary lymphoid organs, in which lymphopoiesis takes place independently of any antigenic stimulus. Normally in the body the lymphocytes only become antigen-responsive after they leave the primary lymphoid organs to seed into the secondary lymphoid tissues. Blood, spleen, lymph nodes, pharyngeal and gut lymphoid tissue, and bone marrow are the secondary lymphoid organs, in which proliferation of lymphocytes normally occurs only in response to specific antigenic stimulus. T and B lymphocytes circulate continuously between the blood and the secondary lymphoid organs, and settle in the latter, or other tissues, only when triggered by an antigen.

In the secondary lymphoid tissues the T and B cells occupy different sites (*Figs 1.3 a, b*). B cells reside in and around the germinal centres of the lymphoid follicles of lymph nodes and spleen, while T cells occupy the paracortical or deep mid-cortical regions of lymph nodes and the periarteriolar regions of the splenic follicles (Malpighian corpuscles). In neonatally thymectomized mice, and in some immunodeficient states in man, these areas can be seen to be deficient in T cells and occupied by macrophages instead.

Plasma cells, which are produced from B cells by antigenic stimulus, are to be found lining the medullary cords of lymph nodes and in the red pulp of the spleen.

Recirculating T and B cells pass through the medulla of the lymph nodes to enter the efferent lymphatics and then, via the thoracic duct, to re-enter the blood-stream. It is possible that the lymph node medulla is the site of T-B cell co-operation.

Recognition of antigen

Both types of lymphocytes recognize antigens by means of specific membrane receptors on their surfaces. The B cell antigenic receptors are undoubtedly immunoglobulins though the exact nature of T cell

Fig 1.3 The T and B cell zones of secondary lymphoid organs

1.3a T.S. of lymph node

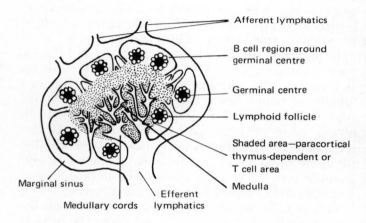

Afferent lymphatics

B cell region around germinal centre

Germinal centre

Lymphoid follicle

Shaded area—paracortical thymus-dependent or T cell area

Medulla

Marginal sinus

Medullary cords

Efferent lymphatics

1.3b T.S. of Malpighian corpuscle of spleen

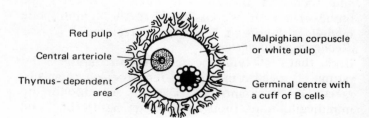

Red pulp

Central arteriole

Thymus-dependent area

Malpighian corpuscle or white pulp

Germinal centre with a cuff of B cells

antigenic receptors is awaiting confirmation. There is a lot of evidence that the antigenic receptors of some T cells are also at least partially, if not fully, immunoglobulins or structurally related substances. It appears that the immunoglobulins of B cells are easily visible by fairly insensitive methods such as immunofluorescence while the immunoglobulins on T cells are scarce and probably differently orientated, and only demonstrable by very sensitive methods such as autoradiography.

Clonal selection (Fig 1.4)

The clonal theory put forward some fifteen years ago by MacFarlane Burnet proposes that during the embryogenesis of lymphocytes, long before any question of antigenic stimulus arises, small numbers or clones of lymphocytes develop, each with surface membrane receptors for a single or very small number of potential antigens. When an antigen gains entry to the body, the few lymphocytes which possess surface receptors exactly or most nearly corresponding to its surface configuration—a matter of only 1 in 10^4–10^5 cells in an unimmunized host—respond to the antigen by differentiation and multiplication. A clone of B cells, when antigenically stimulated, divides and differentiates into plasma cells, which produce humoral antibody, and memory cells, which are responsible for more precise and rapid response to the antigen on future occasions—we may presume that their surface configuration is a more precise and accurate 'fit' with that of the antigen. Hence, each clone which is stimulated leads to secretion of antibodies with appropriate specificity for the antigen which triggered it at the beginning. Each B cell has between 10^4–5×10^5

Fig 1.4 Schematic representation of antigenic stimulation and its consequences

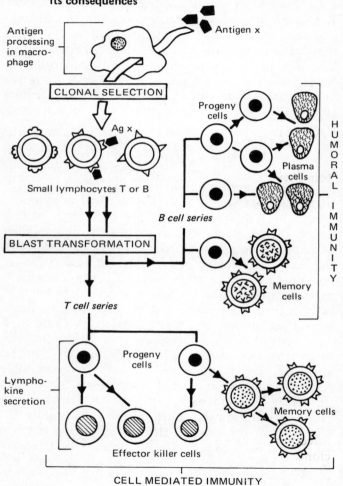

immunoglobulin molecules on its surface through which the antigen is recognized.

The antibody-synthesizing function of the plasma cells—which as mentioned have only a short life—is indicated by the presence within them of abundant rough endoplasmic reticulum.

The T cells also show narrow antigenic specificity similar to that of B cells, i.e. only 1 in 10^4 or 10^5 cells will bind to a particular antigen and the resultant cells of response react specifically with the triggering antigen. When T cells are thus triggered they undergo morphological transformation into 'blast' cells, large primitive cells with small nuclei and highly basophilic cytoplasm rich in RNA. These blast cells differentiate into effector 'killer' cells, and memory cells. The effector killer cells can cause cellular injury to cancer cells, transplant cells, or cells harbouring virus, but they cannot normally deal direct with pathogens.

During the process of proliferation of T cells, large numbers of biologically active protein factors are secreted. Called collectively *lymphokines*, they recruit and activate macrophages to deal with intracellular parasites and micro-organisms.

It is important to realize that a bacterial or a tissue cell has a large variety of distinct antigens on its surface, each variety of which may be repeated on the surface many times; for instance, on the red cells of a group A person there may be 250 antigen A, 300 rhesus antigen D, 290 Lewis antigens, and so on. An infecting bacterial cell, therefore, stimulates many clones of lymphocytes, corresponding to the multiple antigens on its cell surface. Sometimes a bacterium or red cell is, confusingly, referred to as 'an antigen',

although in fact it carries many different surface
antigens which are then referred to as antigenic determinants.

Specificity

Since the original phase of recognition of antigen is
more or less specific, the resultant cells or antibodies
which are being produced are naturally also specific,
the specificity being determined by the overall three-
dimensional configuration of specific regions of the
antigen. The antigen-antibody reaction is thus like
the fitting together of a lock and a key. But just as
one key, while designed for only one particular lock,
may with a slight misfit open another similar lock, so
cross-reactions can occur between antigens and antibodies if there is sufficient partial similarity between
their surface recognition areas. The strength of such a
reaction, and the binding force between the antigen
and the cross-reacting antibody, are weaker than in a
truly specific reaction (*Fig 1.5*).

Memory

Memory is an important distinction between active
and passive forms of specific immunity since it is a
function of memory cells formed during the adaptive
immune response to an antigenic stimulus in a host.
In the case of the B cell (humoral) response, the
progress of this phenomenon is easily illustrated by
measuring the antibody levels produced over a period
of time in response to repeated antigenic stimuli.

In the primary response, antibody can first be detected (if the usual precipitation, agglutination, or
complement fixation tests are used) from the 5th day

Fig 1.5 Cross-reactivity

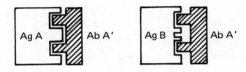

Antibody A' is produced in response to Antigen A, but might cross-react weakly with slightly similar Antigen B.

after the initial stimulus. Peak response is about the 14th day, the antibody level then falling off and becoming low or unrecordable within a month or two.

When a booster injection is given, the body, primed and ready with its larger clone of specific memory cells, responds more rapidly, more strongly, and more lastingly. Much higher levels of antibody appear, within 48–72 hours, and persist for much longer; the quality of these antibodies is more specific; they are less likely to cross-react with other antigens, and antigen-antibody binding is much firmer than in the primary response. A similar memory phenomenon occurs in the cell-mediated response, the cells involved being mainly memory cells from the first response.

The memory cells in both types of immunity have been proved by cell-transfer studies to be small lymphocytes.

1.18

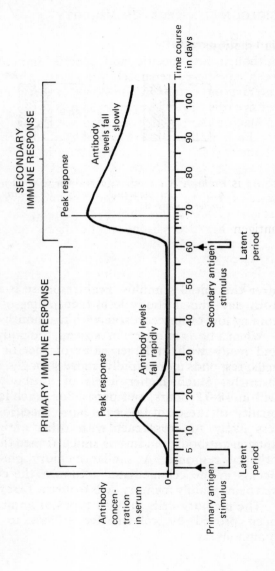

Fig 1.6 Kinetics of primary and secondary immune response to an antigen

Interactions

Although non-specific and specific immunity have been considered separately for clarity, the two forms interact intimately in the body to carry out the defensive role of the immune system.

Macrophages, which are anatomically situated close to the lymphocytes in the lymphoid organs, play an important role in antigenic stimulation. They phagocytose antigen and, while they degrade most of it, some is brought to their surface, probably in concentrated form, to stimulate the immune response. RNA isolated from macrophages containing this ingested antigen has been found to be highly immunogenic and has been termed 'super antigen'. (see *Fig 3.1*).

Macrophages and polymorphs possess specific receptors on their cell membranes for certain immunoglobulins and activated complement factors which enhance their capacity to phagocytose antigen-antibody complexes. Moreover, macrophages are vital as effector cells in cell-mediated immunity also.

The complement system interacts closely with the antibody system, considerably affecting the biological effects of antibody activity.

Thus, the outcome of any infection or insult depends on the fine balance between the activities and interactions of all the different factors of the non-specific and specific immune responses in the host.

Chapter two

HUMORAL ANTIBODY IMMUNITY
AND THE COMPLEMENT SYSTEM

Antibodies
Antibodies are proteins synthesized and secreted by
plasma cells in response to an antigenic stimulus; they
have the molecular properties of immunoglobulins.
The immunoglobulins are glycoproteins composed of
four polypeptide chains. Structurally speaking all antibodies are immunoglobulins but functionally speaking
the reverse is not true, not all immunoglobulins are
functionally antibodies. In most cases the specific
antigen relating with an immunoglobulin is definable
and the immunoglobulin is then called an antibody,
but in those cases where no antigen for it is known, it
is just called an immunoglobulin.

When serum proteins are separated electrophoreti-
cally, the immunoglobulins are found predominantly
in the gammaglobulin fraction, though some are found
in the alpha$_2$ and beta fractions (*Fig 2.1*).

Fig 2.1 Electrophoretogram obtained by UV scanning of paper electrophoresis strip showing diagrammatically the main components of human serum proteins and the three major serum immunoglobulins

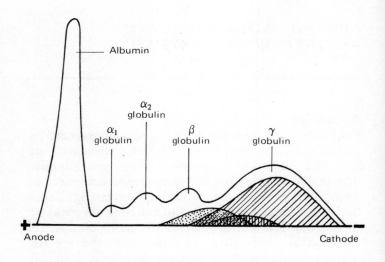

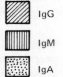

THE IMMUNOGLOBULINS

The four polypeptide chains of the immunoglobulin glycoproteins are themselves formed of aminoacids linked in a particular sequence. Each immunoglobulin molecule consists of two identical heavy polypeptide chains and two identical light chains (so named from their length and molecular weight). Light chains have about 200 aminoacids and a molecular weight of 25 000; heavy chains are twice as long, and therefore twice as heavy.

The heavy chains each have a central flexible 'hinge' section, at which they are linked in pairs by disulphide bonds, and to one half of each heavy chain a light chain is linked, also by disulphide bonds proximally (Fig 2.2a).

The immunoglobulins are not, like haemoglobin or insulin, proteins with a fixed formula and structure. They are a family of proteins, sufficiently alike in their basic structure to be classed together, but with variations which account for class and subclass differences and their varying antigen-binding capacities.

The light chains exist in two different types—kappa (κ) and lambda (λ); 65% of serum immunoglobulins have κ chains, 35% λ chains. The heavy chains are of five main types, known by the Greek letters γ, α, μ, ∂ and ϵ, corresponding to the five major classes of immunoglobulins, IgG, IgA, IgM, IgD, and IgE respectively.

To study the function of the different regions of the complex immunoglobulin molecule, it was first proteolytically digested by papain and pepsin. Papain splits the molecule between the hinge section and the

2.4

Fig 2.2a Diagrammatic structure of IgG molecule

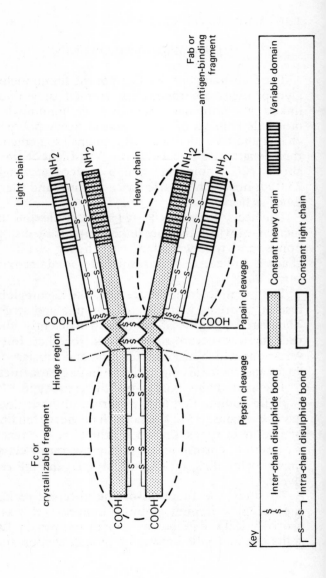

Key

Inter-chain disulphide bond

Intra-chain disulphide bond

Variable domain

Constant heavy chain

Constant light chain

Light chain

Heavy chain

NH2

NH2

NH2

NH2

Fab or antigen-binding fragment

COOH

COOH

Papain cleavage

Hinge region

Pepsin cleavage

Fc or crystallizable fragment

COOH

COOH

Fig 2.2b Diagram showing functions of different domains of an IgG molecule

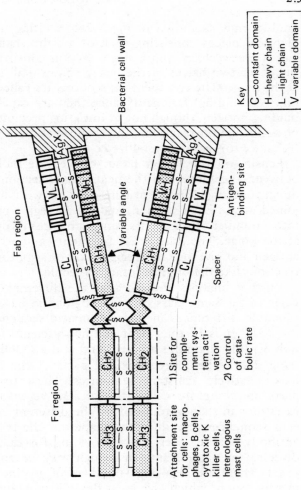

Key

C—constant domain
H—heavy chain
L—light chain
V—variable domain

2.5

Bacterial cell wall

Fab region

Variable angle

Antigen-binding site

Spacer

AgX

V_L V_H V_H V_L

C_L CH_1 CH_1 C_L

Fc region

CH_2 CH_2

1) Site for complement system activation
2) Control of catabolic rate

CH_3 CH_3

Attachment site for cells: macrophages, B cells, cytotoxic K killer cells, heterologous mast cells double end, as shown in *Fig 2.2a*, resulting in two identical pieces consisting each of a light chain and half a heavy chain, and a single section consisting of the other two halves of the heavy chains, still linked at the hinge. The two identical sections are called 'Fab' (antigen-binding) fragments since they are capable of binding antigen, though not of initiating precipitation or agglutination reactions; the single section is called 'Fc', since it is easily crystallized.

Pepsin, on the other hand, cleaves the molecule between the hinge and the heavy-chain section, producing one single fragment consisting of two Fab units joined at the hinge section, and the Fc region broken into a number of fragments, since it has lost its linkage at the hinge. The double Fab fragment can both bind antigen and give rise to precipitation or agglutination reactions like the original intact molecule.

Further analysis showed that the different molecules in the same class of immunoglobulin have considerable differences in their aminoacid sequences at the NH_2 ends of their light and heavy chains (every polypeptide chain has an NH_2 end and a COOH end —*Fig 2.2a*); the more proximal parts of the chains have relatively constant sequences. These terminal parts are therefore called the *variable regions*. The variations in shape produced by the different aminoacid sequences give different shapes to the terminal antibody-binding sites, thus providing for the great diversity of natural antigens which may be encountered. There are also large numbers of glycine units in this region, which give great flexibility in configuration, so that the antibodies can adapt themselves to the antigen shape and make a good fit.

The heavy chains are linked to each other and to their light chains by inter-chain disulphide bonds. Intra-chain bonds divide up the heavy and light chains into several constant domains called C_{H1}, C_{H2}, C_{H3}, and C_L, and one variable domain in each polypeptide chain (*Fig 2.2b*).

The actual antibody-binding site is a groove at the distal end of each F_{ab} segment which can accommodate about three units of the aminoacids or four of the sugars of a linear antigen.

Electronmicroscopic appearance of immunoglobulin

A small divalent antigen, dinitrophenol (DNP), consisting of two identical halves, was used to observe an antigen-antibody reaction under the electron microscope. Reacted IgG molecules showed geometric shapes such as triangles, squares, and pentagons (*Fig 2.3a*), while unreacted antibody molecules were seen to be Y-shaped structures (*Fig 2.3b*).

The small projections at the corners of the molecules in *Fig 2.3a* disappeared after pepsin treatment, confirming that they were the F_c regions of the antibodies.

Biological and physical properties of the immunoglobulin classes

Table 2.1 shows the different biological and physical properties of the five serum immunoglobulins.

IgG, the major component of the serum immunoglobulins, is a monomeric unit with a molecular weight of 160 000, sedimentation rate 7S, and adult serum levels of about 13.2 mg/ml. It is divalent (the

2.8

Fig 2.3 Diagrams of electron micrographs

2.3a Antigen-antibody complexes

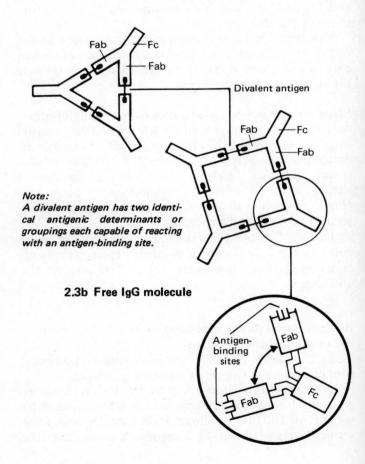

Note:
A divalent antigen has two identi-cal antigenic determinants or groupings each capable of reacting with an antigen-binding site.

2.3b Free IgG molecule

Table 2.1

Biological and physical properties of immunoglobulins

Immunoglobulin	Molecular formular	Physical state	Sedimentation coefficient	Valency (No. of antigen binding sites per molecule)	Molecular weight	Adult mean serum mg/ml
IgG	$\gamma_2 \lambda_2$ $\gamma_2 \kappa_2$	Monomer	7S	2	160 000	13.2
IgA - serum secretory	$\alpha_2 \lambda_2$ $\alpha_2 \kappa_2$ $\alpha_4 \lambda_4, \alpha_4 \kappa_4$ $\alpha_6 \lambda_6, \alpha_6 \kappa_6$	Monomers Dimers Trimers	7S 11–13s	2 4 6	170 000 385 000	1.6
IgM	$\mu_{10} \lambda_{10}$ $\mu_{10} \kappa_{10}$	Pentamer	19S	5–10	900 000	0.9
IgD	$\partial_2 \lambda_2$ $\partial_2 \kappa_2$	Monomer	7-S	2	184 000	0.1
IgE	$\epsilon_2 \lambda_2$ $\epsilon_2 \kappa_2$	Monomers	8S	2	188 000	0.0003

term valency is used in this context to indicate the number of antigen-binding sites on a single molecule).

IgA occurs in two different forms, as a monomer in serum, but polymerized in secretions. The serum form is divalent, the secretory form quadri- or hexa-valent, depending on the physical state of the molecule (degree of polymerization).

IgM, the macroglobulin, is a pentamer, with a molecular weight of 900 000, and thus a valency of 5–10. *IgD* and *IgE* are both monomers, and only present in small amounts in serum.

Fig 2.4 shows the immunoelectrophoretic mobility of the three major immunoglobulins. Normal human serum is placed in the well and subjected to electrophoresis, whereupon, at the pH normally used (8.6), albumin and $alpha_{1,2}$ globulins move towards the anode, beta and gamma globulins towards the cathode. Anti-human globulin from rabbits is put in the trough to diffuse out, and precipitation lines result as shown in the figure. (IgD and IgE are present in too low concentrations in serum to be demonstrable by this method.)

Immunoglobulin G

IgG is the most abundant immunoglobulin in body fluids, forming 75% of the total serum immunoglobulin level. It is equally distributed in the different fluid compartments, hence its importance in defence against diffusing toxins and spreading micro-organisms. IgG antibody response is predominant in the secondary immune response (*Fig 2.5*). To respond to practically all antigens IgG-programmed B lymphocytes require

Fig 2.4 Immunoelectrophoretic mobility of the three major serum immunoglobulins

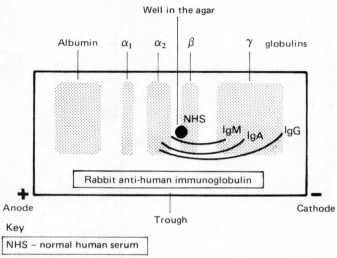

T cell co-operation (the co-operating T cells will usually in future be called 'helper T cells', to distinguish them from other T cells to be mentioned later which do not have this function). The antigen-binding sites on IgG are able to conform better to the shape of an antigen (and therefore bind more firmly) than those of, for example, IgM with the same antigen.

IgG antibodies are highly effective opsonins (substances which promote phagocytosis) since the two major phagocytes of the body, the polymorphonuclear leucocytes and the macrophages, have special receptor sites on their surface membranes for the Fc region of IgG antibodies which promote adherence and thus

2.12

Fig 2.5 The IgM and IgG antibody levels in primary and secondary immune response to an antigen

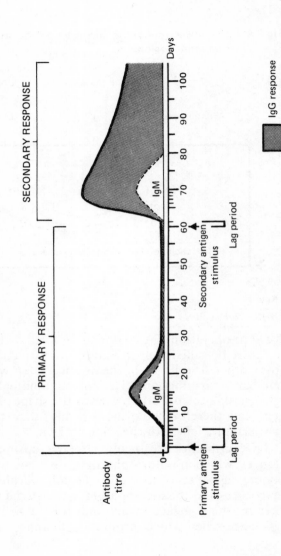

phagocytosis. This is further aided by the complement C_{3b} receptors on macrophages (see later).

Maternal IgG is actively and selectively transferred across the placenta to the fetus and imparts passive protection to the newborn for 4–6 months.

The rate of breakdown of IgG is monitored by a feedback mechanism in the body, in an attempt to keep the serum level normal. In the case of IgG multiple myeloma (see later) the turnover is very high, and some of the important defensive antibodies are broken down as well, so exposing the patient to increased risk of infection.

When involved in antigen-antibody reactions, IgG antibody can activate the complement system and so stimulate its different biological activities, including chemotaxis, vasodilatation, promotion of phagocytosis, and cell- and basement-membrane damage.

IgG antibodies when directed against cell-surface antigen can induce cell destruction through the action of other cells in the body, termed K (killer) cells collectively. This type of killer cell activity is located in the phagocytic cells as well as in the mononuclear, glass-adherent non-phagocytic lymphoid cells. These killer lymphoid cells lack the surface immunoglobulins of B cells or the sheep's red cell receptors of T cells but possess receptors for the Fc region of IgG antibodies; they are probably a special class of lymphocytes and cause cell death of target cells via the Fc-region receptors of the IgG antibodies which coat the target cells. This form of cell damage has been described in transplant rejection and may prove to be important in the autoimmune diseases, in which there are large amounts of IgG-class autoantibodies directed against antigens of the body's own tissues. The role of this phenomenon in cancer immunity is being studied.

IgG is normally found in small amounts in CSF and urine.

Immunoglobulin A

This class of immunoglobulin is found both in serum and in the seromucous secretions of the respiratory, gastrointestinal, and genitourinary surface membranes, and in other secretions such as sweat, tears, saliva, and colostrum. In serum it is monomeric with a 7S sedimentation rate, while in secretions it is in di- and trimeric form with 11–13S rates. Its biological significance in serum *in vivo* is uncertain, although various antibody activities can be demonstrated *in vitro*. Serum IgA cannot activate the complement system; its basic structure resembles that of IgG.

Secretory IgA

The polymeric units of secretory IgA consist of monomer units joined by a short polypeptide chain called a J chain. The polymeric IgA molecule is synthesized by plasma cells in the lamina propria of mucous membranes. On its passage out into the lumen of whatever organ is secreting it the molecule recruits a 'secretory piece' from the epithelial cells (*Fig 2.6*) which is believed to increase the resistance of the IgA to proteolytic digestion after it has been secreted.

The immunoglobulin composition of gastric juice is 80% IgA, 13% IgM, and 7.8% IgG; Burnet has called IgA the 'antiseptic paint' of the mucous membranes. It may function by covering parts of the surface of pathogens and thus inhibiting their adherence to surface mucosal cells and, hence, their entry

Fig 2.6 Diagrammatic structure of secretory IgA

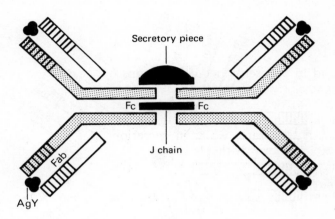

to the body. This possibility is partly supported by reports that about a third of IgA-deficient subjects suffer from recurrent respiratory and gastrointestinal infections. On the other hand an increased incidence of autoimmune diseases has been reported in IgA-deficient subjects.

Secretory IgA can activate the complement system in the presence of lysozyme to kill certain coliform organisms; the biological significance of this observation requires further elucidation.

Immunoglobulin M
This, the largest immunoglobulin molecule (19S sedimentation rate) has a pentameric (5-unit) structure which appears star-shaped on electron microscopy in the free state (cp. the Y-structure of IgG). Its five

Fig 2.7 Diagrammatic structure of IgM

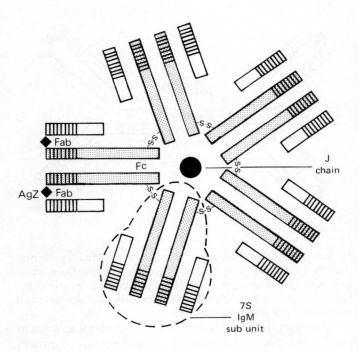

units are joined by a single J chain at the F_c region, and also stabilized by disulphide bonds. Monomeric IgM units (with 7S sedimentation) are found on 10-20% of circulating lymphocytes—these are believed to be virgin B lymphocytes which could either produce

IgM or switch over to synthesize the other immuno-globulin classes on antigenic stimulus. Similar sub-units have also been identified on T cells (see p 2.27).

IgM is usually the earliest antibody response to a primary immune stimulus (*Fig 2.5*) but, since it is short-lived, its presence indicates recent stimulation (e.g. recent infection). The star-shaped free molecule assumes a crablike shape in antigen-antibody reactions.

Most natural antibodies, such as the blood-group AB isoagglutinins, are IgM-type antibodies. Rheuma-toid factor is also commonly an IgM antibody, though it can occur in the IgG class as well. Those antigens which do not involve the thymic-dependent response predominantly stimulate IgM formation.

IgM possesses ten potential antigen-combining sites, but these can only all be effective at once with small antigens; with larger antigens only five sites are effec-tive. The high valency of this molecule gives it a powerful agglutinating and complement-fixing cyto-lytic capacity. It is efficient in reactions with sub-stances such as red cells and gram-negative bacteria which have identical repeated antigenic determinants on their surface, but it is a clumsy molecule for re-action with other substances, for which IgG antibody is better.

This immunoglobulin is essentially limited to the blood-stream, where it is an important protective factor—witness the high incidence of gram-negative septicaemia common in the newborn, who have very low levels of IgM. A raised IgM level in a newborn is a useful indication of intrauterine infection such as syphilis, rubella, toxoplasmosis, etc. A newborn has to synthesize its own IgM, since such a large molecule is unable to cross the placenta from the mother.

Immunoglobulin D is essentially another blood-stream immunoglobulin, present in fairly small amounts. It cannot fix or activate the complement system, and in structure it also resembles IgG. Recently it has been demonstrated on the surfaces of 15% of lymphocytes in the newborn, as against 3% in adults; many of these cells showed the presence of IgM sub-units as well. IgD is not detectable in the serum of the newborn, however, and the evaluation of these findings must be awaited. High serum IgD levels have been reported in kwashiorkor.

Immunoglobulin E is a heat-labile immunoglobulin also normally found only in small amounts in serum, and also similar to IgG in structure. It is attracted to mast cells and basophils. Since mast cells are found mainly in the perivascular tissues, a large proportion of IgE is found perivascularly, sited on these cells, to which it adheres by the Fc region of its molecules.

High serum levels of IgE are found in immediate hypersensitivity reactions (e.g. hay fever, extrinsic asthma, drug allergies) and in helminthic infestations. In the former IgE is playing a *pathogenic* role; no confirmation that it plays any defensive role in the latter has so far been obtainable, however.

IgE deficiency has been reported in a few isolated cases of chronic respiratory infection but not all patients with IgE deficiency get such infections. so it is still uncertain whether IgE ever plays a defensive role. IgE is the same as 'reaginic antibody'.

Fig 2.8 Serum immunoglobulin levels in neonates and children compared to normal adult levels

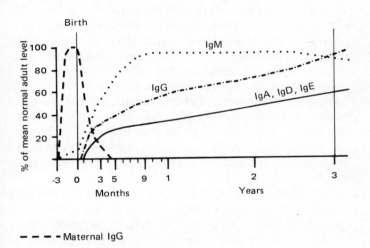

– – – Maternal IgG

–·–·– Infants IgG

Serum immunoglobulins in children and adults

Fig 2.8 shows the development of immunoglobulins in the new born and young child. The rise in immunoglobulins in childhood and the maintenance of these levels may be related to environmental antigenic stimuli, since the levels remain very low in animals reared in germ-free environments. Furthermore, adult serum IgG and IgM levels in underdeveloped countries are higher than those in developed countries, presumably due to more frequent exposure to bacterial and parasitic infections. Serum IgA levels, however, do not vary in this manner.

The low, almost unrecordable levels of IgM in the newborn, the low complement levels, and a sluggish phagocytic action all contribute to the increased susceptibility to gram-negative septicaemia seen in infancy. IgM, however, predominates in the infant and child response to antigens, and adult levels are attained within 9 months of life.

Maternal IgG antibody may be defensive for a new-born on the one hand, but it considerably retards the manufacture of the baby's own IgG in the first 3 months or so of life. The infant's own IgG response matures after 3 months, and this is when vaccination programmes are usually started. Adult values of IgG are reached by age 3.

The serum IgA, D, and E levels begin to rise within a month of birth, and reach about half adult levels by age 3, and adult values at adolescence. Secretory IgA in the saliva and other secretions, however, reaches adult levels in the first few months of life, and can be used as a useful early indicator of any deficiency in the humoral antibody response, for instance in a field survey; attempts to measure infant IgG levels would be interfered with by maternal IgG present.

Multiple myeloma

This disease is classed as a 'malignant monoclonal gammopathy', because it is caused by proliferation of a single clone of plasma cells which secrete large amounts of one type of immuno-globulin with a constant structural composition and physical properties, which moves as a distinct 'M band' on electrophoresis (M for myeloma, not to be confused with IgM—the M band can be in any one of the different classes of immuno-globulins).

Plasma cells normally synthesize light and heavy chains sep-arately, but in correct proportions. In multiple myeloma an excess of light chains is often synthesized, and it is these that overflow through the kidneys as Bence Jones protein. The ex-cess light chains are normally only of one type, κ or λ. The electrophoretic fraction seen in the M band consists of whole immunoglobulin molecules in the serum, formed of the correct proportion of heavy and light chains. These homo-geneous proteins—the whole immunoglobulins in the serum and the free excess light chains in the urine—are useful in the study of immunoglobulin structure and function. They are also useful for preparing pure antisera to the different classes of immunoglobulins and to the light chain fractions.

The cellular events of humoral immuniy (*Fig 2.9*)

Antigenic stimulation of B cells results in the pro-duction of plasma cells which secrete antibodies which react with the stimulating antigen. Function-ally there are two populations of B cells: those which react to antigen with the aid of helper T cells and those which can react independently. The antigens concerned are called thymic-dependent and thymic-independent, respectively.

Most of the biological agents and toxins require helper T cell co-operation to induce a B cell response, i.e. are thymic-dependent. Helper T cell co-operation is especially necessary for IgG antibody response to all types of antigens, and also for the development of memory cells in all humoral antibody responses. Memory cell development is reflected in the lymphoid

Fig 2.9 Diagram of cellular events of humoral immunity

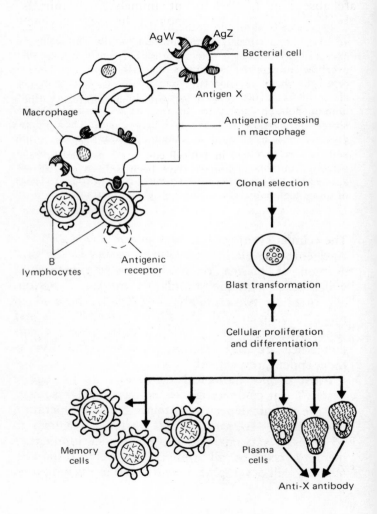

tissues by the development of germinal centres, which are absent in T cell-deficient animals; such animals also have a defective IgG response. The exact mechanism of the co-operation is not clear, but several experimental results and observations suggest the following as a possible mechanism.

The immune system views an antigen in two parts, the carrier, and the hapten; helper T cells are believed to react to the carrier, and then induce B cells to respond to the hapten portion. An accessory adherent cell (probably a macrophage, or a fixed dendritic cell of a lymphoid germinal centre) is an important intermediary in T-B cell co-operation. Helper T cell receptors which bind antigen have been isolated, and these complexes are believed to be released to bind to macrophages in order to stimulate the specific B cells as they come by.

Since the action of this complex in stimulating B cells can be inhibited by antibody to μ heavy chains and to both κ and λ light chains, it is suggested that the helper T cell receptors for the carrier portion of the antigen are IgM sub-units. These are not easily detected by the routine immunofluorescent technique used for B cells (as mentioned in chapter one), possibly because they are very few, or deeply buried.

The common antigens which are thymic-independent are: polymerized flagellin, pneumococcal polysaccharides, gram-negative bacterial polysaccharides, levan, dextran, polypeptide copolymers, etc. These mainly stimulate an IgM response. The IgM-precursor B cells have been reported to possess a receptor for activated complement factor 3 (see below). These antigens could dispense with helper T cell co-operation in two possible ways: (a) by effecting multipoint contact with the B cell surface, and/or (b) by activating the alternate pathway of complement system, releasing activated complement factor 3, which could then act as a second triggering mechanism for the B cells.

Thymic-independent antigens are in fact polymers with a

regularly repeating sequence of antigenic determinants (small antigenic groups) on their surfaces, which favour multipoint contact with B cell surfaces. These two mechanisms may act together to trigger the IgM precursors, but they do not appear effective enough to produce an IgG response or to induce memory cell formation.

Immunoglobulins in clinical medicine

Immunoglobulins are principally used for:

- prophylaxis of certain viral diseases, e.g. rabies, infectious hepatitis, smallpox, and measles;
- prophylaxis and therapy of tetanus, diphtheria, gas gangrene, and snake bites;
- replacement therapy in primary or secondary humoral-antibody-immunodeficiency states to prevent recurrent bacterial infections;
- prevention of maternal sensitization during parturition in cases of maternal-fetal Rh incompatibility;
- prevention of graft rejection in patients with transplanted organs; for this purpose anti-lymphocyte serum, containing antibodies against lymphocytes, is used.

The source of immunoglobulin for most of these purposes is heterologous hyperimmune serum prepared by a planned series of immunizations of animals, but such serum proteins are foreign proteins, and readily induce hypersensitivity reactions on repeated use; if human immunoglobulin can be used the incidence of such reactions is negligible.

Artificial passive immunization, however, should always be followed by active immunization, so as to avoid the anaphylactic reactions which may result on a later occasion if heterologous serum to which the patient has been sensitized is given again.

Immunoglobulins in the tropics

The hypergammaglobulinaemia encountered commonly in the tropics is mainly due to raised levels of IgG, probably in response to repeated parasitic infections.

Raised serum IgA levels are found in patients with pulmonary tuberculosis and in some cases of kwashiorkor.

Variations in serum IgM levels are seen in many tropical conditions; in about half of patients with idiopathic tropical splenomegaly syndrome (TSS) the level is raised, and these patients usually respond better to antimalarial therapy than TSS patients with normal or low IgM levels. Grossly high IgM levels can be found in the serum and CSF in African trypanosomiasis, and a normal level of serum IgM excludes the diagnosis. IgM is normally absent from CSF but it becomes detectable and sometimes considerably raised in bacterial meningitis, trypanosomiasis, and in some forms of encephalitis, but none is detectable in cerebral malaria or cow's urine poisoning; this can be a useful diagnostic point in differentiating these conditions, which commonly affect the CNS in tropical countries.

In kwashiorkor, children with chest infections often show raised levels of serum IgD, although in children who get it below seven months of age serum IgG, IgA, and IgM levels, and antibody response are impaired. On older children the disease has less effect and, as just mentioned, many show raised serum IgA levels, attributed to increased synthesis in the gut wall.

Marasmic children have normal IgA levels.

Antigenic receptors on T and B lymphocytes

As emphasized in the last chapter, the lymphocytes are the immunocompetent cells which can recognize one antigen from another by means of their special surface membrane receptors, called antigenic receptors, and only a few cells in the normal lymphoid population respond to a given antigen, at the most one cell in 10 000 or 100 000 (ref. Clonal selection, p 1.13).

It is now well established that the antigenic receptors on B cells are antibody molecules of the IgM (7S sub-units) and IgD classes, expressed either jointly or singly on the cell surface and having been synthesized by the B cells themselves.

It is found that when such a lymphocyte is antigenically triggered, it proliferates and differentiates to give rise to a whole population of plasma cells. Among this plasma cell progeny may be found all or any of five types of plasma cell, each type with the capacity to secrete one only of the five main immunoglobulins; all the immunoglobulins so produced, however, by plasma cells derived from one original cell have the same variable region, and hence the same antigenic specificity.

Since it is the constant region of an immunoglobulin which determines its class, and the variable region its antigenic specificity, it can be postulated that every B cell contains five genes for the immunoglobulin constant region and one for the variable region. Any given daughter plasma cell may therefore secrete any one (but only one) of the five immunoglobulins but whichever one it is its particular job to secrete, the variable region on it will be identical with those of the other immunoglobulins secreted by its sibling cells.

At what particular stage of cellular proliferation the daughter cells are committed to a particular antibody is still under study, since we start with B cells with only IgM/IgD on their surfaces and end, in any particular immune response, with plasma cells secreting between them any or all of the five classes of immunoglobulin.

The T cell antigenic receptors have not been able to be so clearly defined, since no immunoglobulin molecules can be detected on their surfaces by the common methods which work with B cells. Nevertheless, from the diversity of their antigenic specificity, from clonal selection, and from the genetic standpoint, there is general agreement that the antigenic receptors on T cells are the same as the variable regions of the immunoglobulins of B cell antigenic receptors. The nature of the constant region, and hence the class of immunoglobulin molecule involved, remains in doubt since it is not determinable by the reagents used for B cells. This probably means it is deeply buried in the cell membrane, but it could be of a completely new class which we have as yet no reagents to detect.

THE COMPLEMENT SYSTEM

The complement system (*Figs 2.10, 2.11*) is composed of a complex group of enzymes in the normal bloodstream, some of which have been designated by the

Arabic numerals 1–9.

There are two main ways in which the complement system can be activated. The first, or classical, pathway starts by activating complement factor C_1 and thence the others, more or less in numerical order, until the entire system has been activated. This is the mechanism adopted by antigen-antibody complexes.

The 'alternate pathway' bypasses the first three factors of the classical pathway (C_1, C_4, C_2) and directly activates factor C_3, thereafter following the same terminal stages as the classical pathway. This mechanism is adopted by a variety of substances such as gram-negative endotoxic lipopolysaccharides, inulin, aggregated immunoglobulins, cobra-venom factor, zymosan from yeast walls, and others.

Classical pathway

IgG and IgM antibody are capable of activating the first component of the complement system, factor C_1. This sequentially activates C_4 and C_2, which finally activate C_3—which is the factor present in the largest amount in normal serum. A single complex of activated $\overline{C_{1,4,2}}$, moreover, activates many molecules of C_3, thus producing a multiplying effect.

Some of the activated $\overline{C_3}$ molecules break up and release smaller molecule C_{3a} while C_{3b} remains attached to antigen. C_{3a} functions as an anaphylotoxin and chemotaxin—as the former causing release of histamine and other kinins from mast cells to produce vasodilatation, increased vascular permeability, and bronchoconstriction, etc., while as a chemotaxin it attracts polymorphs and other inflammatory cells to the site as the inflammatory reaction.

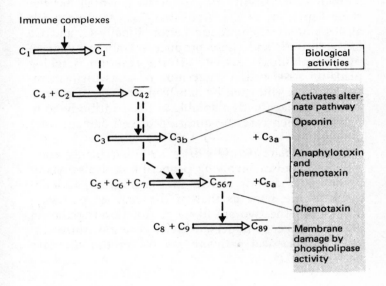

Fig 2.10 Classical pathway of complement activation

Key
C—native complement factor
C̄—activated complement factor

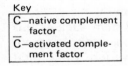

C_{3b} combines with $C_{1,4,2}$ on the target-cell surface and induces adherence of macrophages and polymorphs and thus phagocytosis of immune complexes (*Fig 3.3*). Another function of C_{3b} is to stimulate the alternate activation pathway, thus activating still more C_3 molecules.

Activated $\overline{C_3}$ stimulates in turn activation of $C_{5,6,7}$ (which circulate as a single trimolecule). At this stage a small C_5 fragment, C_{5a}, is released, which has the same functions as C_{3a}. Activated $\overline{C_{5,6,7}}$ trimolecule is also a potent chemotactic factor. Finally C_8 and C_9 are activated, and these produce membrane damage by phospholipase activity. If the reaction is taking place on a red cell, a bacterium, or a basement membrane, these will then be damaged—it may, of course, be taking place with a soluble antigen-antibody complex, in which case the question of cell damage does not arise.

The alternate pathway (*Fig 2.11*) is a highly complex mechanism involving properdin and also many other enzymes not shown in the diagram. Its end-result is the same as that of the classical pathway, and indeed the two are likely to function together in any defensive or hypersensitivity reaction, since C_{3b} from the classical pathway can trigger the alternate pathway.

Inhibition of the complement system
Obviously a complex enzymatic system such as this must have inhibiting enzymes to maintain homoeostasis and prevent premature activation. Congenital absence of such an inhibitor for activated C_1 —called C_1-esterase inhibitor—results in familial hereditary angioneurotic oedema, replacement therapy with the missing enzyme alleviates the recurrent attacks of oedema in this condition, and recent trials with ϵ-aminocaproic acid for prophylaxis have had encouraging results.

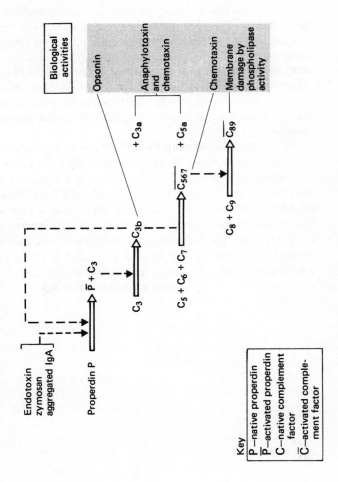

Fig 2.11 Alternate pathway of complement activation

Key
P—native properdin
P̄—activated properdin
C—native complement factor
C̄—activated complement factor

Biological significance of the complement system

It is now recognized that invading pathogens such as bacteria, fungi, viruses, mismatched transfused blood cells, or transplant cells, are attacked by complement once their respective antibodies have identified them, reacted with the invading cells, and activated complement by the classical pathway.

In the early stages of primary infections, however, when no antibodies have as yet been formed, pathogenic material in the body, such as endotoxin or polysaccharides, may activate complement by the alternate (properdin) pathway.

In either case, the biological effect of the activated complement system is to provoke an inflammatory response by increasing blood flow and vascular permeability, attracting inflammatory cells and, finally, encouraging immune adherence and phagocytosis of the pathogens or foreign cells by the inflammatory cells. These are important defensive mechanisms, though in some circumstances they can also result in tissue-damaging or allergic hypersensitivity states (see Chapter seven and summary diagram *Fig 3.3*).

Chapter three

CELL-MEDIATED IMMUNITY

Historical

Early this century the protective part played by serum (humoral) antibodies in defence against many diseases, especially in co-operation with the complement system, was demonstrated; also that protection could be passively transferred from an immune individual temporarily to a non-immune by transfer of serum or some of its constituents. There remained a group of diseases, however, in which passive transfer of serum antibodies was no help, but Chase and Landsteiner in 1942 managed to transfer immunity successfully in some of these diseases by transferring living lymphoid cells from an immune to a non-immune individual.

Meanwhile it had been noted that people with this group of diseases that need cells rather than serum to transfer immunity often showed a delayed skin reaction to intradermal challenge with the appropriate antigen (e.g. old tuberculin in Tb, lepromin in leprosy); they reacted with erythema and induration at the site 24–48 hours after injection; this was called 'delayed hypersensitivity'.

It was now found that transfer of lymphoid cells transferred this delayed hypersensitivity reaction as well; a recipient with a previously negative skin test would develop a positive reaction after receiving immune lymphoid cells.

From these observations sprang the science of cellular immunology which has made such vast strides over the last 30 years.

Definition of cell-mediated immunity

We have seen in the previous chapters that there are two main different forms of immune response, through the T cells and through the B cells; and we have gone into the mechanism of the B cell (or humoral) response. Cell-mediated immunity (CMI) works through the T cells, the thymus-dependent lymphocytes, and its end-results are effected by the lymphoid killer cells which develop from the T cells, and macrophages which are recruited and activated by immune T cells.

The terms 'cell-mediated immunity' and 'delayed hypersensitivity' are, rather confusingly, sometimes used synonymously, but it is better to restrict the latter to the actual tissue damage resulting from the cellular immune response, leaving CMI to cover the entire spectrum of reactions involved in the response, which range from the defensive to the tissue-destructive.

Biological significance of CMI

The biological significance of CMI and T cell function has been clarified by the study of:

- children with congenital absence of the thymus, e.g. DiGeorge's syndrome, Nezelof's syndrome;
- 'nude' mice—mice of a congenitally athymic strain which are also hairless (nu nu strain);
- experiments with neonatally thymectomized mice;

and it has been shown to be involved in:

- resistance to infections
- tumour rejection
- delayed hypersensitivity states
- regulation of the immune system.

Resistance to infections

It appears that in general we are normally dependent primarily on our CMI response for protection against slowly growing intracellular pathogens, while our humoral antibody system protects us from rapidly growing, toxin-producing organisms. And of the two mechanisms of CMI response—forming effector killer cells and activating macrophages—the latter is by far the more important in resisting infections.

Nearly all pathogens, however, have an extracellular phase in which they are susceptible to neutralization or opsonization by humoral antibodies, and in a few other circumstances antibody, in co-operation with the complement system, can also cause target-cell lysis as well as promoting opsonization.

Some pathogens, on the other hand, have subtle methods for avoiding antibody attack in their extracellular phase, e.g. leishmania cause antibodies to aggregate on the surface of their cell membranes, subsequently extruding or absorbing the antibodies without deleterious effect on themselves.

Tumour rejection

It is now generally accepted that actively regenerating tissues are constantly giving rise by mutation to clones of neoplastic cells, and there is clinical and experimental evidence that these abnormal cells are promptly recognized as such by the immune system and eliminated; this function of the immune system has been called 'immunological surveillance'.

Delayed hypersensitivity

This is the state evidenced by tissue damage 24–48 hours after contact with an antigen to which the individual has previously become sensitized. As mentioned, it is often used synonymously with cell-mediated immunity, because tissue damage commonly occurs as a by-product of the CMI response, e.g. the caseation in Tb, the nerve damage in leprosy. In these two examples the tissue reaction, although possibly harmful, is clearly defensive in intent, but there are other situations in which there is no obvious defence purpose in the reaction, e.g. in contact dermatitis and some autoimmune diseases. Transplant rejection may also be included in this latter category, since it is a process which damages tissues which may in fact be desperately needed for the patient's survival.

Regulation of the immune system

We described in Chapter one the co-operative, helper, function of T cells, but they can also have a suppressor function, and the two types of cells (helper and suppressor), each affecting cellular and humoral immunity differently under different circumstances, constitute an immune regulatory system.

Mechanism of CMI
T cells, like B cells, have cell-membrane receptors to recognize antigens but, as mentioned in Chapters one and two, their exact nature is still uncertain. Some suggest they are 7S IgM sub-units, others believe they are genetically controlled structures on the cell surface, the gene responsible being the 'immune response gene' (Ir), located on human chromosome 6 in the same region as the histocompatibility (HLA) genes important in transplant work. (HLA stands for Human Leucocyte Antigen, since leucocytes are richly endowed with these genetically determined antigens.)

Once T cells are stimulated by specific antigen (through macrophage intervention—see Chapter one), they stop circulating, settle in the thymic-dependent regions of the secondary lymphoid tissues, and there undergo firstly blast transformation, and then an active phase of proliferation and maturation.

The first products of proliferation are medium-to-large-size killer cells, which are strongly cytotoxic. These, like plasma cells, are 'end cells'—they cannot divide or mature further and die once their job is done. The later products of proliferation and maturation are small lymphocytes which are only weakly cytotoxic unless further stimulated by specific antigen, in which case they can divide and differentiate further (like memory cells) into more strongly cytotoxic cells.

Cytotoxic cells appear to damage their target cell victims by coming into direct contact with them and

Fig 3.1 Diagram of cellular aspects of induction of CMI

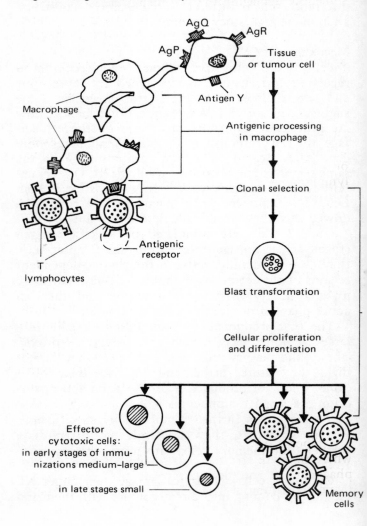

somehow damaging the cell membrane. The number of effector killer cells required to deal with each target cell is quite high, suggesting that the mechanism, *in vivo*, is not very efficient; they can, nevertheless, effectively kill a few neoplastic cells, incompatible transplant tissue cells, and virally infected cells showing viral antigens on their cell membranes.

This direct cytotoxic action is, as we have already said, one way in which the CMI response attacks its target cells, and the other involves macrophages, which are recruited and stimulated by the 'products of activated lymphocytes' (PAL), which we met as lymphokines in Chapter one. T cells stimulated by the specific antigen to which they are sensitized, or by non-specific mitogens (substances causing cell proliferation) have been shown *in vitro* to release the various types of lymphokines listed in Table 3.1. Some of them, e.g. MIF, interferon, TF, have also been detected *in vivo*.

The actual sequence of events in CMI is not established, but it may be deduced from the actions of the lymphokines listed above. Mitogenic and transfer factors released by activated T cells recruit previously uncommitted lymphocytes at the site of the antigen and stimulate them to divide and differentiate, releasing in turn more lymphokines and increasing the inflammatory reaction.

The inflammatory cells, some of them polymorphs but predominantly macrophages, are attracted from the blood-stream to the site of the inflammation where they are arrested and stimulated to accelerated phagocytosis and degradation of the pathogens or target cells (tumour, transplant, or virus-infected cells,

Table 3.1

a) Factors affecting lymphocytes	
Transfer factor (TF)	may transform a local response into a general one by passive transfer of specific immunological information via nucleic acid to uncommitted lymphocytes. TF has been used to transfer CMI therapeutically in some immune-deficient states*
Mitogenic (blastogenic) factor (BF)	induces blast cell transformation in normal lymphocytes or accelerates existing reactions
Cell co-operative or helper factor	increases the number of antibody forming cells *in vitro* and their rate of antibody production
Suppressor factor (postulated)	inhibits activation of B cells or their production of antibodies
b) Factors affecting granulocytes	
Leucocyte chemotactic factor	causes migration of granulocytes (*in vitro*)
Leucocyte inhibition factor (LIF)	inhibits migration of granulocytes
c) Factors affecting macrophages	
Macrophage chemotactic factor (MCF)	causes macrophages to migrate
Macrophage inhibition factor (MIF)	inhibits migration of normal macrophages
Macrophage aggregating factor	agglutinates macrophages in suspension
Specific macrophage arming factor (SMAF)	arms macrophages to attack and kill specific target cells
d) Necrotizing substance	
Lymphotoxin (LT)	cytotoxic for certain cultured lymphocytes, e.g. mouse lymphocytes, HeLa cells[†]
e) Others	
Proliferation inhibition factor (PLF)	inhibits proliferation of cells in culture
Interferon	prevents synthesis of viral proteins in infected cells.

*see p 3.16
[†]a widely used cell line cultured from one original cancer of cervix

as the case may be).

Macrophages act on bacteria by ingesting them into a vacuole in their cytoplasm ('phagosome') into which specialized cell structures or organelles called 'lysosomes' (sacs containing over 25 different acid hydrolases) release enzymes which digest the pathogens.

(Lysosomal hydrolases can also cause substantial cell damage when released extracellularly, as for example in rheumatoid arthritis, in which they are responsible for the joint damage.)

Certain pathogens—streptococci, pneumococci, *H influenzae* e.g.—are normally directly attacked and destroyed by lysosomal enzymes, but certain others, such as *Br abortus*, *S typhi*, *M tuberculosis*, are able to resist lysosomal attack, either by preventing the lysosomes fusing with the phagosomes and releasing their hydrolases, or by secreting some neutralizing substance. Activated macrophages attempt to bypass these escape mechanisms, and the outcome depends on the natural resistance of the pathogen, the infecting dose, and the host species. The destructive capacity of an activated macrophage for any given pathogen varies from one host species to another—this accounts for the natural variation in species susceptibility to any particular pathogen, *M tuberculosis*, for instance, being an exceptionally hardy organism, able to resist attack even by activated macrophages.

Once activated, the activated macrophages are bactericidal or viricidal to any bystander organism, irrespective of the triggering agent; macrophages activated by bacteria have been shown to retard growth of cancer cells in tissue-culture systems as well.

Infections involving CMI

Infections in which CMI features (not necessarily usefully from a defence point of view) include:

● viral—measles, mumps, smallpox, chickenpox/zoster, herpes simplex, cytomegalovirus infection, LGV;

● protozoal—leishmaniasis, toxoplasmosis, Chagas' disease (*T. cruzi*);

● fungal—candidiasis, dermatomycosis, coccidiomycosis, aspergillosis, histoplasmosis, cryptococcosis;

● bacterial—mycobacterial diseases such as tuberculosis, leprosy, Buruli ulcer; brucellosis, salmonellosis, syphilis, tularaemia, meliodosis.

The events in leprosy demonstrate some important aspects of the CMI response. *M. leprae* is an obligate intracellular parasite which initially grows in nerve and muscle tissue, which have no lysosomes. The outcome of repeated or prolonged exposure to leprosy infection depends on the state of immunity of the host. Those with a highly active and vigilant immune system escape clinical disease completely, whereas those with less effective immunity develop one of the clinical forms of the disease.

If the host's T cells are completely unresponsive to leprosy (anergic), the organism is able to multiply freely in the macrophage system; there is no immune response, the lepromin skin test is negative, and the disease takes lepromatous form. If their T cells are partly responsive, however, as shown by a positive lepromin test, then the macrophage system is activated to attack the bacilli, few will be found in the skin and other tissues, and the nerve-destroying granulomatous reaction with which we are familiar in tuberculoid leprosy occurs.

Some patients change from tuberculoid status to lepromatous; in this case their T cells are losing reactivity and becoming anergic. It is worth noting, however, that high levels of humoral antibody against mycobacteria are found in patients with lepromatous leprosy in whom no defensive reaction is taking place.

In considering immunity to viral infections, the phases of infection and reinfection have to be considered separately. Interferon is a naturally occurring antiviral agent synthesized in various tissue cells during viral invasion and secreted (even in non-viral infections) by activated T cells (see Table 3.1). It is very active in blocking virus replication in a cell without interfering with the host cell's own metabolic activities. Since it is a non-specific agent, once its production has been induced, it will function against any other viruses which may invade the tissues. Viruses, however, vary widely in their susceptibility to interferon.

In infections caused by susceptible viruses, recovery from primary infection often coincides with peak interferon levels, while the humoral antibodies and CMI develop later on. Lifelong immunity, however, or reduced severity in reinfections, is a function of the adaptive immune response, whether humoral or T cell-mediated.

In T cell-immunodeficient states in children interferon levels in viral infections are usually the same as in healthy controls, but even so live attenuated viral vaccines such as smallpox or measles are contraindicated, since these children get generalized vaccinia and a disseminated measles-like illness respectively— indicating that such organisms (and the herpes group) are insusceptible to interferon.

Antibodies given immediately after the vaccine, however, are a useful therapeutic weapon which will reduce the severity or abort the attack. Thus serum antibodies are effective and useful in the viraemic phase of a virus infection. Once the viruses have gained entry to the target cells, the CMI response is a better defence.

Neoplastic cell rejection

The high incidence of chemically and virally induced tumours in T cell-deficient animals suggested the concept of immunological surveillance which we have already mentioned. The number of cells involved in this form of immune response is a factor in determining its outcome, however, as the immune system can only deal with a small nidus of neoplastic cells or small metastatic deposits.

Mutating neoplastic cells have new surface antigens ('neoantigens') which the immune system recognizes as abnormal, and which initiate the tumour rejection response. Some of these antigens, and other tumour cell products, are recognizably fetal or embryonic in nature—e.g. the α-fetoprotein secreted by hepatocellular carcinoma cells, which is a useful diagnostic index of hepatoma.

The role of CMI in tumour immunity is not finally proven, and recently some authors have suggested the tumour killer cell may not in fact be from the T cell series at all, but a B cell or an activated macrophage. This idea does not necessarily contradict the earlier observation that there is an increased incidence of neoplasia in T cell deficiency and in immunosuppressed patients, as the T cells may still affect neoplasia by their regulatory effect on the immune system further discussed below.

Delayed hypersensitivity

This term, as we have said, is best restricted to the tissue-damaging reactions, e.g. caseation in Tb, nerve damage in leprosy. Tissue damage may result from

● pathogens and their toxic products;

● killer-cell attack on neoplastic, transplant, or virus-infected cells;

● the necrotizing lymphokine, lymphotoxin, released by sensitized T cells;

● lysosomal hydrolases released by activated macrophages in the process of digestion and degradation of pathogens.

Two or more of these mechanisms may act in co-operation, though the effectiveness of killer cells and lymphotoxin *in vivo* is doubtful, and the lysosomes are probably the most important mechanism in practice. What is more, tissue necrosis often exposes hidden or altered tissue antigens to which the body is not tolerant, so causing autotissue sensitization which may then be responsible for continuing tissue necrosis independently of the initiating immune reaction.

Attempts are being made to dissociate the delayed hypersensitivity (tissue-damaging) aspect of CMI in practice from the defensive parts of the reaction, so that the latter may be therapeutically reinforced without stimulating the former.

In some situations the tissue reaction is purely damaging without any defensive purpose; for example the contact dermatitis due to chemicals, heavy metals, cosmetics, and dyes. Certain insect bites, e.g. mosquitoes, can induce delayed hypersensitivity skin or systemic reactions.

Transplant rejection

Nucleated tissue cells possess genetically determined membrane antigens called HLA antigens, just as red cells have ABO/Rh antigens. In identical twins such antigens are identical, and siblings have some in common. HLA antigens can be detected by serological means and are called 'serologically defined antigens'; there are other cell-membrane tissue antigens against which, unlike the SD antigens, it has proved very difficult to raise antibodies, and these can only be recognized by tests employing lymphocytes, wherefore they are called 'lymphocyte-defined antigens'.

These two systems play an important part in the outcome of transplantations: if there is genetic compatibility between donor and recipient the transplant will survive, but if the two are incompatible it will be rejected. T cell-mediated immunity is largely, but not solely, responsible for rejection, and the immunosuppressive therapy used in transplant patients is aimed at damping down T cell function.

We see therefore that where neoplasia is concerned immunotherapy aims at immunopotentiation; in transplant work it is aimed at immunosuppression.

Regulation of the immune system

We have already discussed the role of helper T cells in promoting the B cell response to the majority of biological antigens, and there is a T helper effect in CMI, essential for formation of T memory cells, as well. As mentioned briefly earlier, however, it has been found that T cells can also have a suppressive action, on both the humoral and cell-mediated responses. Antigen-specific T cells thus regulate T and B cell responsiveness, with effect ranging from complete stimulation to complete suppression, though in most cases the result is somewhere in between these two extremes.

T cell suppressive actions have been reported in:

● some forms of immunological tolerance (specific non-responsiveness);

● antigenic competition (one antigen interfering non-specifically with the immune response to another. Reducing the number of T cells reduces the likelihood of such an effect);

● prevention of autoimmune diseases (experiments indicate these arise from lack of suppressor T cells);

● regulation of IgE response (believed to be inhibited by suppressor T cells; large amounts of IgE are synthesized if they are absent. Helper T cells have also been shown to be involved in the IgE response).

B cells also influence the immune system in two ways:

● under certain circumstances sensitized B cells can signal normal or sensitized T cells to act as suppressor cells;

● a factor has been isolated from the serum of patients with enlarging disseminating cancers which interferes with cell-mediated cytotoxicity by all types of killer cells in the body including those which kill by attaching themselves by their cell membrane Fc receptors to the free Fc ends of IgG-target cell complexes, and exerting their killer action through the IgG antibody without actually coming in contact with the target cells. This factor has been shown to be an immune complex of tumour antigen/host antibody; thus a B cell product—antibody—can suppress the tumour immune reaction by inhibiting the final effector mechanism, cytotoxicity (see *Fig 6.1*).

Similar interference with cell-mediated cytotoxicity by immune complexes may be important in promoting survival of parasites especially adult forms of helminths.

Although macrophages may also have some suppressor effects, there is conclusive evidence that they have a helper effect, both in the induction of the immune response and in the effector mechanisms of both humoral and cellular immunity, as we have already seen.

Thus interactions between cell and cell, and between cells and cell products, play an important role in the regulation of the immune system. The possibility of additional factors such as hormones (and through them nervous factors) also having an influence on the immune system also has to be borne in mind.

Transfer factor in therapeutics

Transfer factor is a non-immunoglobulin molecule in T cells which, as we have said, can generalize a local reaction to antigen by activating lymphocytes in parts of the body remote from the original reaction site. It can also be administered to non-sensitive recipients, in which case it confers on them cell-mediated immunity and delayed hypersensitivity and converts their lymphocytes, *in vivo* or *in vitro*, to a specific antigen-responsive state. TF can be prepared by various methods from leucocyte homogenates. It is also, of course, as we have seen, released *in vivo* during the CMI response.

Physical properties

● small dialysable molecule of molecular weight less than 10 000; hence non-immunogenic and with little danger of

causing serum sickness;
- heat-labile, but stable indefinitely if stored at 4°C;
- non-immunogenic;
- a short protein chain linked to 3–4 RNA bases, the biological activity being in the chain;
- negligible danger of contamination with HB_SAg.

Biological properties
Some workers claim TF activity to be specific; others believe it works by augmenting the T cell pool in the body. There is evidence to support both these theories.

The exact mechanism of its action is ill understood, and it may also act on the macrophages. Its effect develops within 8-12 hours of administration and persists for a period of a few months to two years, as judged by skin reactivity (e.g. with tuberculin in the case of Tb transfer factor).

Clinical uses
TF has been tried by many workers in a large number of small pilot studies, each involving only a few patients. Larger double-blind trials have now been started, but their results are not yet published. The main indication for use of TF is deficient or suppressed CMI, as judged by skin test reactivity and other now-available *in vitro* tests on the patient.

TF for therapeutic use in infections is mainly obtained from leucocytes from donors with a strong delayed-type skin reactivity to the relevant organism; in neoplasia, *in vitro* tumour cytotoxicity tests are used to assess the suitability of donor leucocytes, which are usually either obtained from family members or from patients who have recovered from a

Fig 3.2 Classification of immunodeficiency states

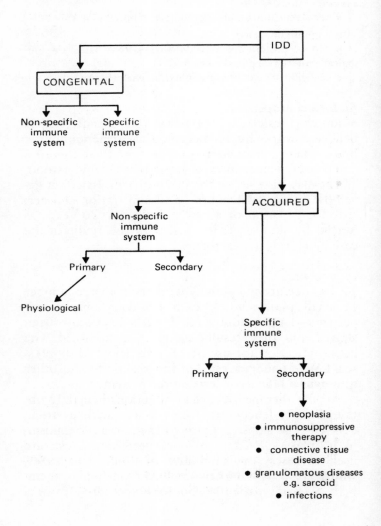

similar malignancy.

The immunodeficiency states, of which the aetiology is outlined below, will largely be covered in a later chapter. Here we are mainly concerned with the use of TF in acquired secondary immunodeficiency. The results of extensive work in this field may be summarized as follows:

Diseases in which clinical improvement has been reported from TF therapy

- progressive primary Tb resistant to chemotherapy
- disseminated coccidiomycosis
- disseminated mucocutaneous candidiasis
- generalized vaccinia and vaccinia gangrenosa
- severe measles with interstitial pneumonia
- chronic aggressive hepatitis (mostly associated with HB$_S$Ag
- sarcoidosis
- juvenile rheumatoid arthritis
- certain neoplasms—
    malignant melanoma
    nasopharyngeal carcinoma
    carcinoma of breast
    osteogenic sarcoma.

Diseases in which TF therapy has been tried, so far unsuccessfully

- lepromatous leprosy
- rheumatoid arthritis
- SSPE (subacute sclerosing panencephalitis)
- acute leukaemia
- Hodgkin's disease
- alveolar sarcoma of soft tissues.

The clinical results of trials of transfer therapy in multiple sclerosis have not been reported yet.

It is to be noted that clinical improvement following transfer therapy may be associated with reversal of abnormal *in vitro* tests, and development of, or return of, skin reactivity, but that the opposite does not always apply, e.g. many of the cases of lepromatous leprosy in which it has been tried developed lepromin skin sensitivity and *in vitro* leucocyte responsiveness without any clinical improvement in their leprosy.

Summary diagram
Fig 3.3 summarizes diagrammatically the essential points of the co-operation between the body non-specific and specific immune mechanisms which have been discussed in the past three chapters.

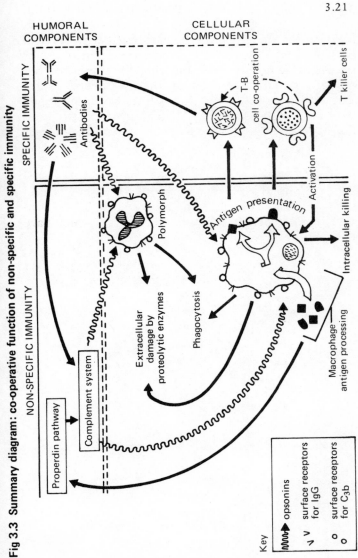

Fig 3.3 Summary diagram: co-operative function of non-specific and specific immunity

3.21

HUMORAL COMPONENTS

CELLULAR COMPONENTS

SPECIFIC IMMUNITY

Antibodies

T-B cell co-operation

T killer cells

NON-SPECIFIC IMMUNITY

Antigen presentation

Activation

Polymorph

Intracellular killing

Extracellular damage by proteolytic enzymes

Phagocytosis

Complement system

Properdin pathway

Macrophage antigen processing

Key

opsonins

surface receptors for IgG

surface receptors for C3b

Chapter four

IMMUNITY TO BACTERIAL AND VIRAL INFECTIONS

There are two major aspects of the subject of immunity to infections to be considered, the pathogen with its subtle ability to enter and survive in the host, and the immune system of the host which struggles to limit the infection or its harmful products and so maintain the constancy of the internal milieu of the body.

The ultimate outcome of the contact of any infectious agent with the host may be one of the following:

● *infection without disease* This state includes latent or silent infections, as well as symbiosis, in which the organism remains silently in the body without causing any clinical symptoms or signs of its presence. An alteration in host immunity may, however, change this state into disease at any time;

● *infection with disease* Here there are two main possibilities: on the one hand a disease state (i.e. clinical effects) may be attributable directly to a pathogen and its toxic products; on the other hand effects may mainly result from the hypersensitivity of the host immune response to the pathogen and its products. Thus the host immune response may either be purely defensive against infection or, at other times, be itself the immediate cause of the pathological manifestations.

This chapter is devoted mainly to the discussion of the ways in which pathogens evade the non-specific and the specific immune mechanisms of the host, but a few facts related to immunity to infections are recapitulated at the end of the chapter; the hypersensitivity state is dealt with in Chapter seven.

PATHOGENICITY AND VIRULENCE OF BACTERIA AND VIRUSES

Pathogenic micro-organisms may be broadly classified into:

● those which interfere with *non-specific* immune processes such as
  i) the phagocytic system
  ii) interferon
  iii) tissue barriers.

● those which interfere with *specific* immune processes, such as those related to
  i) the immunogenicity and pathogenicity of the organisms and their products
  ii) the time course of the primary immune response
  iii) suppression of the immune system
  iv) other escape phenomena from immunity.

Non-specific immune processes
Phagocytic system
Some micro-organisms establish an infection in the body by evading the phagocytic system by possessing or secreting antiphagocytic substances which either

prevent phagocytosis, or are toxic or lethal to phago-cytes. Yet other organisms survive and multiply intra-cellularly by interfering with other processes involved in phagocytosis.

Antiphagocytic substances

● the capsules of *Streptococcus pneumoniae*, klebsiellae, *Haemophilus influenzae*, *Bacillus anthracis*, and *Yersinia pestis* are antiphagocytic and allow unchecked extracellular multi-plication;

● protein A of *Staphylococcus aureus*, protein M of *Streptococcus pyogenes*, and the pili of pathogenic gonococci are also antiphagocytic. Coagulase from staphylococci produces a fibrin deposit on the bacterial surface which may also act similarly;

● many pathogenic viruses are also poorly phagocytosed by macrophages though the exact antiphagocytic element res-ponsible has not yet been identified.

Phagocytotoxicity

Myxoviruses, vaccinia, and measles are cytotoxic to macrophages. Similarly many pathogenic bacteria secrete exotoxins and enzymes which are leucotoxic, e.g. *Staphylococcus aureus* secretes leucocidin which can kill polymorphs.

Survival and proliferation within phagocytes

Some organisms such as pneumococci and *Haemo-philus influenzae* are readily destroyed intracellularly once phagocytosed but *Brucella abortus*, salmonellae, and mycobacteria avoid intracellular death in macro-phages by preventing the fusion of the phagosome and the lysosome. When macrophages are activated by cell-mediated immunity, however, brucellae and salmonellae become susceptible to intracellular killing; mycobacteria, however, are very hardy and sometimes survive even within activated macrophages. Recently some reports have suggested that a combination of an antibody with activated macrophages may be more successful in killing this hardy organism intracellularly.

Similarly, some viruses are readily killed by macrophages while others are resistant and proliferate unchecked in the body.

Interferon

Interferon is a nonspecific antiviral agent which is secreted by almost all tissue cells when infected by viruses. It acts intracellularly by inhibiting the synthesis of viral proteins by the infected cells without interfering with general cell metabolism. When it is excreted extracellularly, it prevents viral infection of neighbouring cells. Many viruses, however, can evade interferon-induced non-specific immunity, as witness the occurrence of lethal measles, or generalized vaccinia following smallpox vaccination, in patients with immunodeficiency of T cells but normal interferon secretion. Other viruses theoretically susceptible to interferon, such as pathogenic influenza viruses, induce only a poor interferon response in the tissues compared with the response to non-pathogenic strains.

Under some circumstances pathologically altered host tissues, e.g. neoplastic lymphoma cells, lose the ability to produce interferon and are thus easily invaded by and support other viruses; these may then be wrongly thought to be oncogenic viruses rather than the 'passengers' they actually are.

Tissue barriers

Tissue spreading, damaging, and pathogenic factors can be produced by pathogens. *Clostridium welchii* and *Streptococcus pyogenes* secrete hyaluronidase, lecithinase, collagenase, and haemolysins, which promote intercellular spread of toxins and pathogens through the extracellular matrix.

Specific immune components
Immunogenicity and pathogenicity
The pathogenic part of any organism or toxin may be different from its immunodominant or antigenic (*Fig 4.1*, A, D) part; and antibodies produced by the body against the dominant region may not neutralize the toxic properties of the organism or toxin. Laboratory tests may show positive agglutination or flocculation reactions and yet there may be no neutralization of toxic effects in biological tests or in the patient. An immune response to these dominant antigens is of defensive significance, however, since it enhances phagocytosis either by an opsonic effect or by activation of macrophages, both of which can effect immune resistance.

Most organisms are also poor immunogens while present in small numbers and thus they can establish themselves in the host before the immune system is

Fig 4.1

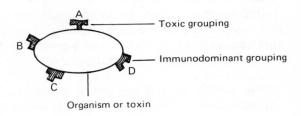

Toxic grouping

Immunodominant grouping

Organism or toxin

alerted to respond. The exotoxins secreted by
C diphtheriae, *Cl tetani*, and *Cl botulinum* cause
lethal disease by prompt attachment to target cells
even when only present in tiny amounts. The toxins
are present in sufficient amounts to be biologically
active in causing disease but insufficient to induce an
immune response, as may be the case with tetanus.
Some toxins may be poor immunogens even when
present in large amounts in the body.

Time course of the primary immune response

The lag period in primary immune response is 4–5
days in an acute infection caused by potent immunogenic pathogens and may be longer still in the case of
poorly immunogenic organisms or toxins. The dose of
a pathogen necessary to trigger an immune response
also varies with its immunogenicity and route of
entry and rate of multiplication. The minimum time,
however, is 4–5 days and the peak response occurs
later still.

During this comparatively lengthy lag phase, the
pathogens gain a preliminary advantage over the host
since the generation time of most pathogens causing
acute infections is very short; the pathogen is thus
well established in the body before enough antibody
or activated macrophages and polymorphs are recruited to deal with it. In chronic infections, such as
with mycobacteria, the time period and dynamics of
host response are different and we see a granulomatous reaction occurring simultaneously with a repair
process.

One of the greatest advantages conferred by prior
immunization is the shortening of the host response

lag period to a day or so. Also many vaccines or toxoids used in active immunization include adjuvants which increase their immunogenicity and ensure a good immune response even to an otherwise poorly immunogenic organism or toxin.

Immunosuppression
The common observation of a negative Mantoux reaction following BCG, in the presence of active tuberculosis, or in patients with or after measles, whooping cough, chickenpox, or infectious mononucleosis, has long been accepted as evidence for the concept of immunosuppression. This concept is supported by *in vitro* tests on blast transformation of lymphocytes which is inhibited by measles and rubella viruses.

The exact mechanisms involved in this phenomenon are not fully unravelled but possible contributory factors are that T cells in man have receptors for measles, influenza, and para-influenza viruses and B cells for EB virus and the arboviruses; also herpes simplex replicates in macrophages. These viruses may thus interfere with the biological activities of the cells involved in the immune system. Similarly, *B pertussis* infection can affect the recirculation pattern of lymphocytes between blood-stream and lymphoid tissues; this may affect the memory cell population necessary for the Mantoux test.

The practical implication of this depressed immunity is that such patients can get a prolonged non-healing viral infection, a latent viral infection, a carrier state, develop a flare-up of latent pulmonary tuberculosis, or get other secondary bacterial infections.

The common problem of secondary bacterial infection following viral infections may be related to the finding of depressed macrophage phagocytic activity in mumps, measles, influenza, and coxsackie infections.

Other escape phenomena from immune mechanisms

There are essentially two types of escape mechanisms, those affecting the non-specific immune factors as mentioned above and those involving specific immune factors.

Antigenic drift, whereby a virus changes its antigenic character and so evades the protection conferred on the individual by infection with a previous variant, is a well-known phenomenon with the influenza and common cold viruses. It results in episodic epidemics. Continuous mutation is an inherent property of all living things including bacteria and viruses; the fittest mutant, which can best evade antibiotic action and the host immune reactions, is the one which survives and propagates. *Borrelia recurrentis* causes relapsing fever by continuous antigenic variation actually occurring during the infective episode in the host. Every febrile relapse is caused by the emergence of a new antigenic variant of the organism, resistant to the antibody stimulated by the previous one.

Many bacteria may persist in the body following an infection in 'L' or long forms which have lost their surface coat and its associated antigens, so that the antibodies directed against these surface antigens are ineffective in eradicating the infection. Similarly, measles virus spreads in the CNS from cell to cell by incomplete nucleocapsids unaffected by the presence of antibodies directed against the capsular antigens of measles virus. Other viruses such as herpes evade lethal antibody effects by spreading directly from cell to cell in the CNS without entering the extracellular space.

There is a distinct possibility that the immune complexes formed by pathogen antigen and the host antibody during an infection or during treatment (see *Fig 6.1*) may block the lymphocyte receptors or macrophage phagocytic system, as happens in the case of disseminated neoplasia. This process could also affect the course of disease in patients.

Immunocompetence of host

It is obvious from study of immunodeficient and immunologically suppressed patients that the immunological integrity of both non-specific and specific immune components is vital for defence against infections. While the majority of the so-called non-pathogenic organisms are rendered non-toxic by competent non-specific immune mechanisms of the body such as the phagocytes, complement system, lysozymes, interferon, and so on, co-operation between antibodies (mainly IgM and IgG type) and the complement and kinin systems is necessary to ensure an inflammatory response which attracts phagocytes to the site of disease; secretory antibodies from the mucous membranes may also hinder the entrance of pathogens into the body.

The exact mechanism of defence in each individual infectious disease is far from being fully elucidated but, in general, pyogenic infections are controlled mainly by humoral antibody; diffusing toxins are also neutralized by IgG antibodies which equilibrate effectively in the extravascular and intravascular compartment and enhance prompt phagocytosis through the Fc receptors for IgG on macrophages and polymorphonuclear neutrophils (ref. p 2.11 and *Fig 3.3*).

Cell-mediated immunity operates against slowly growing intracellular bacteria and against many rapidly proliferating virus diseases such as smallpox and measles. In bacterial infections CMI mainly acts through activated macrophages, while in viral infections direct target-cell killing of virus-infested cells also occurs and this may help to limit the infection (ref. p 3.11 and *Fig 3.3*).

Local CMI in the mucosal surfaces may also play an important defensive role in tuberculosis, as does systemic CMI in leprosy, brucellosis, smallpox, and measles.

Prior immunization with toxoids, or attenuated or killed organisms, is successful in preventing many bacterial and viral diseases such as tetanus, diphtheria, typhoid, whooping cough, plague, Tb, polio, smallpox, yellow fever, measles, and German measles. In the case of BCG, however, the protection against Tb is only partial.

IMMUNIZATIONS AGAINST
BACTERIAL AND VIRAL DISEASES

The concept of immunization against infectious diseases stems from the observation that persons who recover from certain diseases such as smallpox and measles are immune to further infections by the same agents. Apart from resulting from overt attacks of disease, immunity may also be produced by repeated subclinical infections with many organisms, for example diphtheria and pseudomonas bacilli, and individual strains of influenza virus. It would be dangerous, however, to wait for such natural events to occur in a whole population, and many of the potentially lethal diseases of childhood, and some of adult life, have been dramatically controlled by the artificial immunization programmes routine in most countries.

The three aspects of immunology relevant to prophylactic immunization are study of the immunizing agents, the vaccines—their type, potency, source; of the immunocompetence of the host, to determine the optimum times for vaccinations; and of unwanted reactions to vaccinations.

Vaccines

There are three main kinds of vaccine in general use: live attenuated organisms, killed inactivated organisms, and toxoids (detoxified toxins) (Table 4.1). In some cases, such as polio, measles, and plague, both live attenuated and killed forms are available.

The type of vaccine used determines the number of doses required initially to induce satisfactory immunity. Attenuated live organisms multiply in the host producing a massive input of antigen, so that usually only a single dose is needed to induce long-lasting immunity, while killed vaccines or toxoids require two or more doses to induce effective immunity, one priming and one or more reinforcing doses, and poss-

Table 4.1

Type of vaccine	Examples
Live attenuated organisms	Smallpox, polio, measles, anthrax, BCG for tuberculosis, rubella, yellow fever
Killed organisms	TAB for typhoid/paratyphoid, pertussis, typhus, influenza, measles, polio
Toxoids	Diphtheria, tetanus

ibly 'boosters' later in life. (The fact that three doses of live oral polio vaccine are normally given appears at first sight to contradict what has just been said, but these are given because the vaccine contains three different strains of virus and in a significant number of people only one or two strains establish themselves successfully at each feeding; to obtain the best results in as many people as possible, three feedings are best.)

Killed bacterial organisms or toxoids have certain advantages: a much larger quantity can be used for immunizing than would be lethal if unmodified toxin or live organisms were being used—for example one-hundredth the amount of diphtheria toxoid used for immunization would be lethal if it were active toxin; secondly, such vaccines can be purified by physico-chemical methods to remove unwanted substances and products, reducing the possibility of side effects and hypersensitivity reactions; thirdly, killed vaccines and toxoids cannot do any serious harm to children with congenital or acquired immunodeficiency, for whom live vaccines are absolutely contraindicated.

Adjuvants, such as the alum salts used in triple vaccine, enhance the primary and secondary immune response, even if only given in the first dose and not in the reinforcing doses. The pertussis vaccine component of triple vaccine also acts as an adjuvant for diphtheria and tetanus components. Other factors such as the route of vaccination, the metabolic fate of the antigen, and the purity and stability of the vaccine under field conditions all play a role in the outcome of vaccination programmes in practice.

Duration of protection
Certain vaccines induce almost complete, long-lasting protection, e.g. smallpox and polio vaccines, and triple vaccine. Others such as BCG induce substantial and fairly long-lived, but not complete, immunity; in spite of this, the routine use of BCG has virtually eradicated miliary tuberculosis and tuberculous meningitis. Yet other vaccines, such as TAB (typhoid, paratyphoid A and B), give rather temporary and partial protection and require to be boosted at relatively short intervals if cover is to be kept up, as may be desirable in hyperendemic areas.

In general vaccines may be divided into two groups according to their uses: (1) those used for routine immunizations in general medical and public health programmes (see Table 4:2), and (2) those used for special groups such as travellers, or workers in certain hazardous occupations.

Routine immunizations
The immunization schemes used in tropical countries are a little different from those usual in temperate

countries; in the tropics it is important to provide early protection for children against many of the diseases encountered, since their morbidity and mortality are mostly more serious and occur at a younger age than in temperate climates. It is also desirable to get on with as many injections as possible before an infant is 'lost'.

Vaccines for special groups

● TAB is of some protective value against typhoid and paratyphoid; this may justify its use in high-risk school-age populations, but not as a routine in the general population. It is also used for travellers.

● Cholera vaccination is still required for travel to a few countries; under international health regulations it should be repeated every 6 months for continuous cover. The protection it gives against clinical cholera is both limited and short-lived, and it does not control carriers at all.

● Plague vaccine is recommended for field workers at risk, such as geologists, biologists, anthropologists, or surveyors working in the bush in an endemic area, and perhaps for sewage workers. It gives quite good protection although boosters are required at fairly short intervals.

Host immunocompetence

The immunological apparatus is not fully competent functionally at the time of birth and only matures gradually during infancy.

Non-specific factors

The macrophages show a poor and slow chemotactic

Table 4.2

Vaccine	No of doses & interval	Primary course Tropics	Temperate countries	Boosters	Comments
BCG	1	Birth to 3 mths	10–13 yrs	—	70–80% protection (might possibly be lower when given at birth). Highly protective against Tb meningitis and miliary Tb
DPT	3 at 6–8 wks intervals	3–6 mths	usually 6 mths +	DT only school entry and 8–12 years	90–100% protection from potent, unexpired vaccine
Oral polio	″	″	″	School entry	″
Measles	1	6–9 mths	1–2 yrs	After age 1 if first dose given before 1 year	Maternal antibodies may interfere with the take at 6 mths, hence the need for booster
Smallpox	1	1–2 yrs	Not recommended routinely except for health workers	8–12 yrs (do not give within 3 wks of DT)	Necessary for travellers

response which may well influence antigenic processing and the quality of the specific immune response. Some of the complement properdin system levels are lower than in adults, also contributing to the poor chemotactic and opsonic performance of macrophages in neonates. Immune adherence, and the lytic capacity of neonatal serum, however, are relatively normal.

Specific immunity

The initial, IgM, response to most potent antigens is adequate in the newborn, but the switch-over to the IgG response occurs much more slowly than in adults. Maternal IgG antibodies, which survive in the infant for 6–9 months, also interfere with and retard the infant's IgG response to various stimuli. This interference is mainly antigen-specific, e.g. maternal measles antibody interferes with measles vaccination in the infant, and maternal polio antibody with *inactivated* polio vaccine (but not with live oral polio vaccine, as the maternal IgG does not reach the gut to interfere with colonization of the gut epithelium by the modified polio virus). It is therefore some months before the infant can mount a satisfactory IgG response and, ideally, routine vaccinations should not be started before the age of six months. The immunogenicity of a vaccine also affects the immune response, however, and highly immunogenic triple vaccine, for example, can be given satisfactorily at a fairly early age.

Delayed hypersensitivity and cell-mediated immunity may, as with humoral immunity, show a variable response depending on the immunogenicity of the antigen used. Skin graft rejection, for instance, may be normal but the results of contact sensitization with DNCB are less uniform (see p 10.17). A fair degree of protection has been reported following BCG given at birth, however, with very few reports of dissemination of or untoward vaccine reactions, and this justifies its use at birth in the tropics.

Reactions to vaccinations

Three types of reaction may be encountered but it should be emphasized that the protection afforded by the routine childhood immunizations far outweighs the chance of a serious reaction, especially in the tropics.

Infection

Live attenuated vaccines can cause clinical infection, either from error in preparation, testing, or dose of the vaccine, or in the immunodeficiency states.

Hypersensitivity reactions

These may be due to the vaccine itself or to impurities it contains. Any of the four kinds of hypersensitivity reaction (see Chapter seven) may be caused by, particularly, some of the tissue proteins in the tissue culture in which viruses have been grown. Rarely, neuroallergic (encephalitic, myelitic, neuritic) CNS reactions may occur; the vaccines which caused this type of reaction most often were the older types of rabies vaccine.

Toxic reactions

These are relatively common with the enterobacterial

vaccines (TAB, cholera) due to the presence of toxic substances. Such reactions may be reduced by further purification of the vaccines.

Chapter five

IMMUNITY TO PARASITIC DISEASES

Parasitic diseases of man may be broadly classified into the following categories:

● *protozoal infections* caused by unicellular organisms which multiply in the host resulting in a large antigenic stimulus in spite of there being only a small primary inoculum; typical examples are malaria, trypanosomiasis, leishmaniasis, amoebiasis, and toxoplasmosis;

● *metazoal infections*, which include helminthic infections caused by multicellular parasites which do not generally multiply in the host so that the antigenic load stimulus is related to the worm burden in the body.

Resistance to parasitic infections resembles that to bacterial and viral infections, though environmental factors such as climate, habit and habitat of host, customs, diet, and occupation play a much more important role with parasites than with micro-organisms. A warm moist climate, poor hygienic conditions, and overcrowding all favour parasitic infection.

Non-specific immune response

Besides environmental factors, innate or non-specific natural immunity plays a very important role in resistance against parasites in man; only 20 protozoal species out of the 8000 that exist in the universe, for instance, can infect man.

Racial and genetic factors also contribute to resistance, e.g. American negroes are more resistant to *P vivax* and hookworm infection than their white counterparts. The susceptibility of white population to *P vivax* may be attributed to the presence of Duffy blood group antigens on RBC which are believed to be used as receptors by the parasite to gain entry to the red cell to cause malaria. Again, the change in the internal environment of the red cell caused by the present of haemoglobin S in the sickle cell trait, or by G6PD deficiency, confers partial resistance to *P falciparum* malaria. Similarly some humoral factor in the serum of man kills the cattle strain of *Trypanosoma brucei* while the human strains are well supported. The macrophages of leishmania-resistant animals kill the parasite while cells from susceptible animals cannot. Innate resistance may thus be considered of prime importance in determining the pathogenicity in many parasitic infections.

Adaptive immune response

There has long been controversy as to the existence of an adaptive immune response in parasitic infections because, in most, little clinical protective immunity develops. There is now abundant evidence, however, that human parasites are immunogenic and do sensitize the host, producing clinical immunity which can be classified into three main types, depending on the quality of the memory response induced.

● *sterilizing immunity* The only convincing example of this in man is cutaneous leishmaniasis caused by *L tropica*, where the host who recovers from the infection is usually immune to future attack by the parasite: there must be long-lasting memory response in this disease;

● *no effective immunity* Here previous infection does not result in any immunity to future infection by the same organism. Examples are human African trypanosomiasis, human visceral leishmaniasis, Chagas' disease, intestinal amoebiasis, and hookworm infections. In all these conditions an antibody response is demonstrable but it has no protective effect against future attack: there appears to be no effective memory response in these diseases;

● *non-sterilizing concomitant immunity* In this type some resistance to subsequent challenge exists in the presence of low-grade parasitaemia in the host. This clinical state, which has been called 'premunition', occurs in malaria, schistosomiasis caused by *S mansoni*, and ascariasis: such infections induce a short-lived memory response.

The parasite evolves many different ways of evading the host immunity and so manages to maintain a low degree of parasitaemia although the host is relatively immune to fresh infection by the same parasite. These methods of evasion are aptly called 'escape mechanisms'; they may take many and diverse forms as listed below.

Escape mechanisms of parasites

● *Antigenic variation* This phenomenon is typically described in African trypanosomiasis (see below) and in some animal malarias, but other examples may also be classed under the same heading. For instance, the infective phase of a parasite may be antigenically quite different from its other stages and so an immune response to one stage may be ineffective against others. This is seen in malaria, where the protective antibody is directed against the merozoites and has no effect on the sporozoites which are the stage infective to man. In other parasitic conditions, such as amoebiasis, the tissue-invading protozoa lose their surface antigens altogether.

● *Antigenic disguise* This phenomenon was shown to occur with the adult worms and late stages of schistosomula in Rhesus monkeys. The host blood group antigens (A or B) cover the adult worm, thus hiding the parasitic antigens from attack by antibodies and/or cells. This phenomenon probably occurs in man.

● *Interference with immune induction* The parasite, its products, or immune complexes resulting from parasitic infections, can affect the T helper cells or macrophages, or induce formation of T suppressor cells which could all interfere with immunological stimulation of the body. Malaria, for example, has been associated with a poor antibody response to tetanus toxoid and *Salmonella typhi* antigen O, and with an impaired cell-mediated immunity.

● *Interference with immune effector mechanisms* by affecting humoral antibody, cytotoxic T cells, macrophages, polymorphs, and eosinophils. Protozoa such as entamoebic trophozoites avoid phagocytosis by producing factors which degranulate and kill the host's leucocytes. Secretion of large amounts of soluble antigens by parasites could quench antibody and cell receptors peripherally before they reach the original parasite. The last two mechanisms could also account for the secondary bacterial infections which commonly complicate parasitic diseases.

● *Anatomical location* Some parasites, as in malaria, evade immune resistance by entering cells (RBC) where they are inaccessible to the antibody. Others, such as *Toxoplasma gondii*, *Trichinella spiralis*, and echinococci form cysts round themselves which are impermeable to antibodies and sensitized cells.

A few salient features of some parasitic infections

are summarized below.

Malaria
There is good evidence for the existence of concomitant immunity in malaria. Passive immunity is effective in preventing lethal malaria in the baby of an immune mother during the neonatal period. The protective antibody has antimerozoite activity which blocks the entry of merozoites into red cells. A low degree of parasitaemia is maintained in malaria in spite of this antibody by a combined effect of one or more of the following evading mechanisms: antigenic variation, immunosuppression of the inductive or effector phase, and the intracellular site of some stages of the cycle. In malaria-endemic regions, repeated fresh infections could also contribute to a continuing low-grade parasitaemia.

African trypanosomiasis
This disease induces formation of large amounts of IgM antibodies in serum and CSF which is a useful diagnostic criterion. A finding of normal IgM level in serum is against the diagnosis of African trypanosomiasis. Similarly CNS involvement is unlikely in the absence of IgM antibodies in CSF. This parasite-induced IgM protective antibody reduces parasitaemia. A small number of parasites, however, change their antigenic make-up to another variant which is resistant to the original antibody, and this variant starts proliferating, giving rise to a fresh wave of parasitaemia, and so on until the patient dies from the lethal disease or from secondary infection. This parasite is very well adapted to the host and evades immune resist-

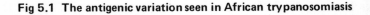

Fig 5.1 The antigenic variation seen in African trypanosomiasis

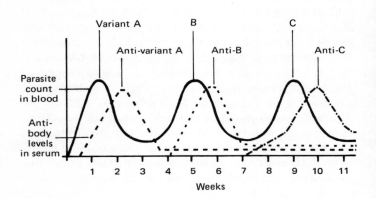

ance by sequential antigenic variation (*Fig 5.1*).

Intestinal schistosomiasis caused by *S mansoni*
In this disease there is evidence of concomitant immunity which limits fresh infection with more cercariae, possibly by antibody-mediated cell cytotoxicity which may involve immune IgG antibody and a killer cell such as the eosinophil. The adult worms residing in the host blood vessels provide a continuous immune stimulus for this lethal antibody but evade its action on their own surface antigens by covering themselves with host blood group antigens.

Whether the same immune resistance and host-evading mechanism is employed by other strains of schistosomes is not known.

Intestinal helminths

This is a large group including nematodes such as *Enterobius vermicularis, Trichuris trichiura,* ascaris, hookworm, and *Strongyloides stercoralis*, as well as the cestodes, which include the tapeworms. A fair amount of work has been done on animal models but it cannot be extrapolated to man since the results in different species of hosts vary considerably. Some animals develop sterilizing immunity, others partial immunity, and some no immunity at all.

In man, premunition has been reported in ascaris, *Taenia saginata*, and *Trichinella spiralis* infection. Some innate natural immunity, as described for American negroes and hookworm earlier in this chapter, is reported in all the helminths. Hookworm infection, however, fails to stimulate any adaptive (specific) immune resistance in man. Eosinophilia and raised levels of IgE reaginic antibodies occur with most of the intestinal helminths but their role in immunity is still ill-understood. It has been suggested that an IgE antibody reaction with worm antigens may trigger off mast cell degranulation, and so release vasoactive amines which may cause worm expulsion from the gut by stimulating contraction of intestinal muscle, but this hypothesis awaits proof. Eosinophilia probably results from the same mechanism as in Type 1 hypersensitivity (see Chapter seven).

In summary, it can be seen that our knowledge of immune resistance to parasitic infections in man is fragmentary and incomplete; more so since extrapolation from animal work to man can only be made with great caution.

Chapter six

CANCER IMMUNOLOGY
TRANSPLANTATION IMMUNITY

CANCER IMMUNOLOGY

Realization that immunity plays a part in cancer arose from various observations.

● There have been a few reports of spontaneous regression of malignant cancer of the breast, melanoma, Kaposi's sarcoma, extra-abdominal neuroblastoma, and so on;

● incidental findings at autopsy of cancerous changes of neuroblastoma, and cancers of thyroid and prostate are about 40 times the clinical incidence of these tumours;

● the incidence of malignancy in the congenital immunodeficiency states is about 10 000 times that in normal controls;

● the incidence of malignancy in immunosuppressed transplant patients is also much higher than normal, as mentioned later in this chapter,

● some autoimmune diseases, such as pernicious anaemia, rheumatoid arthritis, and Sjögren's syndrome, also have an increased association with malignancy;

● in animal experiments it has been shown that neonatally thymectomized mice have an increased susceptibility to chemical and viral carcinogens, which abnormally easily induce tumours in them; tumours transplanted to such mice also survive abnormally long.

Immune surveillance

Burnet therefore postulated the phenomenon of 'immune surveillance', by which is meant that the immune system constantly detects and destroys abnormal clones of cells as they arise in the body, thus preventing them from becoming established. This hypothesis is still subject to confirmation for if such surveillance was completely effective, cancer would never occur: as it does occur, we have to seek an explanation.

Escape of neoplastic cells

From animal experiments there is good evidence that chemical and viral carcinogens are often immunosuppressors as well as carcinogens and the additive effect of these two actions on the host may be responsible for malignancy. Moreover, the cell kinetics of such tumours are such that the tumour grows faster than the immune system responds to its presence; the primary immune response is slow, and the tumour is often established to an extent with which the immune system cannot cope by the time it reacts

Fig 6.1 Blocking effects of soluble immune complexes on the killer cells in the body

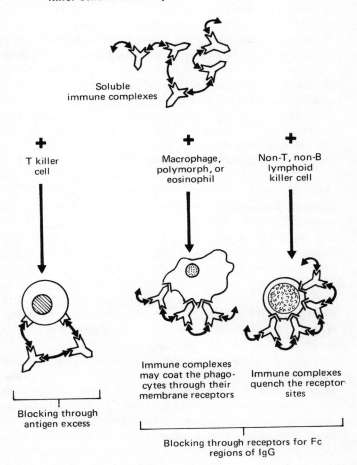

significantly (the immune system can only deal effectively with a small number of abnormal cells, not with a large mass).

It is also becoming increasingly realized that once a tumour is established and has reached a certain size it produces large amounts of tumour antigen. This may combine with the body's protective antibodies to form immune complexes (called 'blocking factors') which appear to block immunological toxicity to cancer cells, at least *in vitro* and probably *in vivo* as well. The presence of large amounts of tumour antigen in the circulation also blocks cytotoxic cells directly, as well as by immuno-complexing with them (*Fig 6.1*).

Immunological rejection of tumours
An immunological reaction against a tumour only occurs if there are foreign antigens on it which are not present in the parent tissue from which the tumour has arisen. Such tumour-specific antigens do occur, and have been termed 'neoantigens'.

From experimental tumour-induction in animals it has been shown that the neoantigens of all tumours produced by a particular *oncogenic virus* are the *same*, regardless either of what tissue the tumour is arising in, or in what host it is induced.

Tumours induced by *chemical carcinogens*, on the other hand, have *different* neoantigens for each tissue in which the tumour arises, i.e. two tumours induced at different sites in the same animal will have different neoantigens; tumours induced in different strains or species of animals by a given chemical carcinogen also have different neoantigens—there is no cross-reactivity between chemically induced tumours as there is with

Fig 6.2 Neoantigens of virally and chemically induced tumours

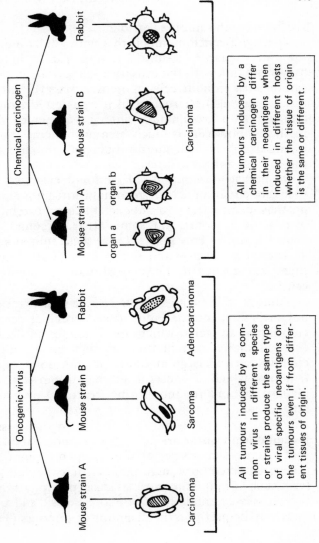

All tumours induced by a common virus in different species or strains produce the same type of viral specific neoantigens on the tumours even if from different tissues of origin.

All tumours induced by a chemical carcinogen differ in their neoantigens when induced in different hosts whether the tissue of origin is the same or different.

virally induced tumours (*Fig 6.2*).

The significance of this is that with virally induced tumours immunity against a tumour can be induced by vaccination with the causative agent or by immunization with tumour cells; moreover, passive immunization may also be successful if transferred from an immune to a non-immune animal. Neither of these methods, however, is much help in inducing tumour immunity against chemically induced tumours, since the tumour antigens differ.

In human tumours there is some evidence that there are common neoantigens in Burkitt's lymphoma, postnasopharyngeal carcinoma, bladder carcinoma, osteogenic sarcoma and some other sarcomas, and neuroblastoma. This suggests that these tumours may be caused by viruses and search for a viral cause for them may eventually be successful and of use in prevention.

Tumour cells may shed or secrete other antigens not present in normal adult tissues, such as carcinoembryonic antigens, which are often found on fetal cells. Similarly, certain tumours such as chorioncarcinomas secrete large amounts of chorionic gonadotrophins which are useful in the diagnosis of the malignancy and for monitoring treatment and recurrence.

Immunodiagnosis

The macromolecules secreted or shed by tumour cells can be detected by a large number of immunological tests such as radioimmunoassay, agar precipitation, or the cross-over immunoelectrophoresis test, and these tests may be useful in the diagnosis of tumours (Table

Table 6.1

The macromolecules secreted by tumours which are used in immunodiagnosis

Macromolecule from tumours	Benign occurrence	Malignancies
Carcinoembryonic	Fetal alimentary system (100%) Fetal plasma (100%) Some inflammatory conditions of respiratory and g-i tract (20–50%)	Pancreas (92%) Colon and rectum (73%) Bronchus (72%) Liver (67%) Other g-i tract (60%) Breast (52%) Neuroblastoma (80–100%) G-U tract (30–40%) Leukaemia and lymphoma (25%)
α-fetoprotein (αFP)	Fetal liver (100%) Fetal plasma (100%) Plasma during pregnancy (1.2%) Hepatitis plasma (0.2%)	Hepatoma (30–80%) Teratocarcinoma (30–80%) Chorioncarcinoma (30–80%)
γ-fetoprotein	Fetal gut, thymus, spleen, placenta	75% of all malignant tumours
Fetal sulphoglycoprotein (FSA)	Fetal g-i tract Peptic ulcer mucosa and secretions	Gastric carcinoma (in gastric secretions)
α_2-H-fetoprotein	Fetal liver and plasma Cirrhosis plasma (40%)	Childhood neoplasms (50–90%) Miscellaneous adult neoplasms
βS-fetoprotein	Fetal liver (not serum) Cirrhosis plasma	Hepatoma (50%)
Leukaemia-associated antigen (LAA)	Fetal tissues Fetal plasma	Miscellaneous leukaemias (30%) Hodgkin's disease

Note: Besides being a diagnostic aid, the assays for these substances are a useful guide to the effectiveness of treatment and to early detection of recurrence or metastasis.

6.1).

Oncofetal (or carcinoembryonic) antigens may be either an intrinsic cell component or may be excreted as a cell by-product. The patient does not usually produce autoantibodies against these carcinoembryonic antigens and they are therefore believed not to take part in protective cancer immunity.

It is interesting to note that certain naturally occurring tissue antigens, such as the blood group antigens A, B, and H, disappear in certain tumours once they metastasize, and this criterion may be of use in assessing tumour spread and deciding on treatment policy.

Effector mechanisms in resistance to cancer

The immune response to tumour-associated neoantigens is quite complex and so the results of *in vitro* tests should only be related to the situation *in vivo* with caution. The various mechanisms of cytotoxicity (see also *Fig 9.2*, p 9.11) are:

● *cytotoxic antibodies* These operate by interaction either with the complement system or with certain mononuclear cells such as:

a) macrophages

b) B cells

c) non-T, non-B lymphoid killer cells.

Complement-mediated cytotoxicity is particularly effective in the leukaemias and against circulating metastatic cells from solid tumours. Cell-mediated toxicity may be of importance in rejection of solid-tumour cells.

● *cytotoxic T cells* from animals with small localized tumours have been shown to be specificially cytotoxic to tumour cells and to be capable of inhibiting tumour growth *in vitro* (as shown with neuroblastoma). Tumour-sensitized T cells also exert anti-tumour activity through macrophages by several mechanisms:

a) by secreting a lymphokine called SMAF (specific macrophage-arming factor) which causes macrophages to exert a specific cytotoxic effect on tumour-cell cultures *in vitro*;

b) by non-specific macrophage activation through MIF and MCF secreted by T cells which enhance tumour-cell cytotoxicity non-specifically; this may be the main rationale for the partial success which has been achieved with BCG immunotherapy;

c) by lymphotoxin secreted by sensitized T cells, which can be cytotoxic to tumour cells; recently B cells have also been shown to secrete lymphotoxin.

Although various types of cytotoxicity that can occur and be demonstrated *in vitro* are known, those related to cancer immunity specifically *in vivo* remain an unresolved puzzle so far, and the whole situation is complicated by the blocking factors in serum mentioned above.

As will be noticed, the mechanisms of cytotoxicity believed to be involved in cancer immunity, transplant rejection, and autoimmune diseases are similar, though the immunological treatment of cancer involves boosting these mechanisms, while that of rejection and autoimmune disease involves suppressing them.

Immunotherapy

Immunotherapy for cancer has gained some acceptance because the principle seems promising, but the actual results achieved so far are hardly striking. The first and absolute requirement for immunotherapy to succeed by itself is that the tumour be very small—in the range of 10^8 cells in man; otherwise other forms of cancer therapy are still the first line of treatment. In various applications, to be mentioned below, immunotherapy may be effective, however, in enhancing the effect of other forms of therapy when combined with them.

Non-specific stimulation
Immunopotentiators such as BCG, pertussis vaccine, and *Corynebacterium parvum*, have been used, but none of them are standardized agents and their use is limited by development of local ulcers at the site of injection. BCG therapy has been tried locally into skin tumour nodules, however, with complete regression in some cases.

Specific immunotherapy
Passive cell-mediated immunity (the transfer of immune lymphocytes obtained from a patient who has had complete regression of a similar tumour) has been tried in some advanced malignancies such as melanoma (as adjuvant therapy) and has produced a few remarkably long remissions; passive antibody transfer has not been widely used and has not had much success in the few terminal disseminated cases in which it has been tried (in addition to regular chemotherapy).

Assisted immunization
Transfer factor therapy in malignancies was discussed in Chapter three.

'Immune' RNA therapy for animal cancers has gained popularity but has not been attempted in man. Immune RNA is a subcellular fraction obtained from immune lymphocytes from an immunized animal, and it mediates both humoral and cellular immunity. Immune RNA can also be used across different species and still be effective, i.e. that prepared from rabbit lymphocytes is effective in tumour-bearing rats.

Specific active immunization
Specific therapy uses the patient's own tumour cells, or those from another patient with a similar tumour, inactivated by radiation, which ensures non-viability but does not affect cellular integrity and antigenicity. About 10^9 cells are given at three different sites once a week.

Mathe was the first to report encouraging results with this method, in acute lymphoblastic leukaemia, though he also used BCG. Other workers' results have not been so impressive, however. Recently this form of treatment has been reported to lengthen remissions in acute myeloid leukaemia as well.

Immunotherapy has been widely tried in malignant melanoma but, although local BCG therapy into tumours has met with some success, specific immuno-therapy has not produced very encouraging results.

TRANSPLANTATION IMMUNITY

Organ or tissue transplantation is the treatment of choice in medical conditions in which an organ is irreversibly damaged, or in congenital defects of vital organs. The extent to which this method is available, however, has been greatly hampered by the noncooperation of the recipient, whose body often endeavours to reject the donor tissue.

The terminology of this subject has changed, and to avoid confusion we shall first give the new and nowadays generally accepted terms, and their meanings, alongside the older terms (Table 6.2).

It was observed very early on that autografts and isografts were practically always successful while allografts were usually rejected. Graft rejection is an immune reaction mediated by lymphocytes and their products; it was first recognized by Medawar, who showed that the reaction was specific and with a memory which resulted in accelerated rejection if a

Table 6.2
Terminology

New (generally accepted)	Old	Meaning
Autograft	Autograft	Using one's own tissue for grafting
Isograft or syngeneic graft	Isograft	Genetic identity between the donor and recipient, e.g. monozygotic twins
Allograft	Homograft	The donor and recipient are of the same species though genetically non-identical
Xenograft	Heterograft	The donor and recipient are of different species, e.g. pig and man

graft from the same donor was transplanted a second time into a recipient.

Blood transfusion is the commonest allografting procedure used in medicine today, and the consequences of a mismatched transfusion are well known. The rejection of solid organs and tissue grafts is somewhat more complex and not yet fully understood.

Immunogenetics of transplantation

In all mammals, all nucleated cells carry on their surface membranes transplantation antigens which are the products of a cluster of linked genes—the 'major histocompatibility complex' (MHC)—on one chromosome pair. These gene products play the main role in allograft rejection if genetic incompatibilities exist.

The MHC and its gene products have been well studied in mice; at least 31 genetic loci controlling the transplantation antigens are known, of which most are of rather weak immunogenicity and so relatively of minor importance in rejection. The strongest complex is known as the H2 region, and consists of many genes which have been fully mapped. In man, the MHC is believed to be as complex as in mice, though only the strongest part of the complex is so far identified; this is known as the HLA system (Human Leucocyte locus A).

The HLA system is composed of two main types of cell-membrane antigens, the serologically determined SD antigens, and the lymphocyte-determined LD antigens. The SD antigens induce antibody production if an incompatible graft is transplanted. SD antigens of paternal origin on fetal cells induce antibody formation in mothers antenatally—this is the commonest source of antisera used for tissue typing.

SD antigens (Fig 6.3)
Each human chromosome pair 6 has three loci for SD antigens, called SD A, B, and C. For each locus there are large numbers of alleles which result in at least 35 different variants; if an individual is heterozygous for all three loci, then he has six different SD antigens on his cells—three derived from the maternal and three from the paternal chromosome—and this allows at least 18 000 different possible combinations.

LD antigens
The LD antigens are detected by the mixed lymphocyte reaction (MLR) which is outlined in Chapter ten. It has proved exceedingly difficult to raise antibodies against the LD antigens in practice, and this has retarded progress in understanding the variants that can

Fig 6.3 Major histocompatibility complex of human chromosome 6

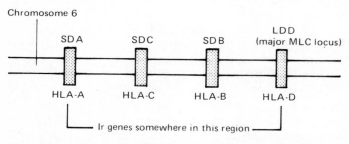

Note: The old (SD and LD) nomenclature is given above each locus and the new (HLA) below.

exist in this system, though a few of them are known. Again, there are at least two loci for LD antigens, a major and a minor, so named for their immunogenicity, incompatibility at the major locus being more lethal than incompatibility at the minor.

Incompatibilities between weaker histocompatibility antigens are relatively easily controlled by the immunosuppressive therapy which is usually given when transplanting an allograft, but incompatibility affecting the stronger antigens invariably results in graft rejection in spite of immunosuppressive therapy.

Choice of donor
1) Since an identical twin is rarely available as a donor, a sibling with complete HLA matching is the best donor.

Any child born to the couple in *Fig 6.4* would have one of the four patterns of genes for the three SD loci shown. Thus there is a 1 in 4 chance that any siblings will match, and a 1 in 2 chance that they will have at least a 50% match if not complete identity for SD antigens. As the family increases the chances of the last-born matching one of its predecessors of course increase. On the other hand, while there is always a chance that two siblings will not share any genes, a parent must always have 50% genetic identity with his or her child for both the SD and LD loci.

The LD loci are closely linked to the SD loci in the MHC region and hence, amongst siblings, compatibility of SD antigens usually correlates with that of LD antigens, except in rare cases when a break has occurred during meiosis (gamete formation) at the MHC region.

Fig 6.4 Genotype of HLA region for SD loci in a family

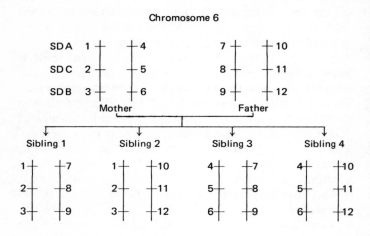

2) A cadaver (usually unrelated) is an alternative donor source. In European populations the results of transplantation support the view that using SD-compatible donors gives better results and reduces the severity of any rejection crisis, but American figures contradict this, which possibly reflects differences in genetic background.

It is also desirable that the blood groups of donor and recipient match.

Privileged sites
There are certain avascular tissues for transplantation of which HLA typing is not needed, such as the cornea, provided the recipient has not had eye disease causing vascularization of the cornea. Vascularization

of the grafted cornea results in a rejection reaction and cloudiness.

Bone and vessel grafts to be transplanted are first killed by boiling; in this form they merely provide a supportive frame for the host tissues.

Immune mechanism of allograft rejection

Cadavers are still by far the commonest source of organs for transplantation in practice. The excellent co-operation between various tissue-typing centres in Europe allows the selection of the best HLA match for a particular patient. Even when the donor and recipient are siblings, however, and HLA-matched, it has proved important to use immunosuppressive therapy to prevent chronic graft rejection, which still occurs as a late complication even in the presence of HLA compatibility; this implies that other transplant antigen systems also exist of which we are as yet unaware but which play some role in the outcome of transplantation.

There is some evidence that the SD and LD antigens which can be typed may not be the ones actually inducing and promoting transplant rejection, but may be closely linked to them in some fashion by linkage of the genes in the MHC region of chromosome 6.

It is widely accepted that primary tissue graft rejection of all solid tissues and organs except haemopoietic tissue (bone marrow) is a delayed hypersensitivity phenomenon mediated by the T cells.

Secondary rejection phenomena can be either T or B cell-mediated. Immunosuppressive therapy is more effective in suppressing T cells than B cells, however, and therefore chronic rejection is often antibody- and complement-mediated (i.e. the result of activity by the less effectively suppressed B cells).

The non-B, non-T killer cells may also inflict cyto-toxic damage through IgG antibody (see Chapter two, p 2.13).

Presensitization of a recipient with circulating anti-bodies against the HLA or ABO antigens of the donor results in hyperacute rejection of the graft as soon as circulation to it is fully established, a matter of hours. It used to be believed, since rejection of skin trans-plants in mice could not be produced by injecting the antibodies, that skin graft rejection was entirely a cell-mediated phenomenon. It is now known, however, that if fresh complement is injected with the anti-bodies, skin transplants are also immediately rejected.

In the case of cadaver organs, the state of autolysis of the organ and ischaemic changes must also play a major part in the future function of such an organ, but *in vivo*, in the recipient, there is no easy way of distinguishing graft failure due to these causes from immune rejection.

HLA antigens and diseases

Various studies have demonstrated a significant associ-ation between some diseases and HLA antigens while others show a weaker association and yet others none at all. In acute lymphatic leukaemia the survival rate and prognosis have also been correlated with certain HLA antigens. Diseases showing significant correlation with HLA antigens are shown in Table 6.3.

Little or no such correlation has been reported in rheumatic fever and breast cancer.

Positive associations have been reported between

Table 6.3
Correlations between HLA antigen and specific diseases

Diseases	HLA antigens
a) Diseases showing a strong association	
1) Ankylosing spondylitis Reiter's syndrome Nongranulomatous uveitis Salmonellal and *Y enterocolitica* arthritis	HLA-B27
2) Myasthenia gravis Coeliac disease Dermatitis herpetiformis Chronic active hepatitis	HLA-A1, HLA-B8
3) Multiple sclerosis	HLA-A3, HLA-B7, HLA-D7a
4) Paralytic poliomyelitis	HLA-A3, HLA-B7
5) Acute lymphatic leukaemia	HLA-A2, HLA-B12
6) Juvenile diabetes mellitus	HLA-B8, HLA-BW15
b) Diseases showing a weaker association	
1) Psoriatic arthritis Juvenile rheumatoid arthritis Asbestosis	HLA-B27
2) Systemic lupus erythematosus	HLA-B8, HLA-BW15
3) Hodgkin's disease	HLA-A1, HLA-B8, HLA-BW35
4) Graves' disease Addison's disease	HLA-B8
5) Australian aboriginal carriers of HB antigen	deficiency of HLA-BW15

LD determinants and multiple sclerosis and diabetes of juvenile onset. The presence of certain LD and SD antigens has also been correlated with earlier onset, poorer prognosis, or faster progression of disease, as for example with acute lymphoblastic leukaemia and HLA-A9.

Significance of the association

The significance of the association of SD and LD histocompatibility antigens with diseases is not thoroughly understood but correlation of the findings with animal work suggests that certain genes of immune response called Ir genes, present in and around the SD and LD regions of the chromosome, are probably related to the increased susceptibility. Either they may preferentially allow certain viral infections to occur or by controlling the immune response to the foreign agent or autoantigen involved they may affect the pathogenic mechanisms involved in the diseases.

Certain other genes within or in the neighbourhood of the MHC also affect the general immunological competence of a person. A close linkage of haplotype HLA-A10 and B18 and deficiency of complement factor 2 has been reported. A similar link has been described with factor B of the alternate pathway. Recent reports on mice models strongly suggest that the gene for synthesis of C_4 is really within the H2 region of chromosome 17. Hence, in man, C_2 and factor B of the alternate pathway are regulated by some of the genes of the MHC gene complex.

The small region of the major histocompatibility complex thus consists not only of the genes of SD and LD membrane antigens but has also other genes responsible for regulating immune responsiveness and affecting predilection for certain diseases, and yet others which affect some of the components of the complement system in serum and thus contribute to the general immunocompetence of the host.

Chapter seven

HYPERSENSITIVITY STATES

The introduction of a particular antigen into a host is followed by the induction of an immune response, and upon second contact with the same antigen the response occurs more rapidly and with greater vigour. This secondary immune response, which is exquisitely immunologically specific, may have either a protective effect, or be tissue damaging, or be a combination of the two, as we saw in Chapter three on cell-mediated immunity.

Definition
The terms *hypersensitivity* or *allergic state* refer to an altered state of the host, whether or not this is beneficial in the long run, following exposure to an antigen, whereby subsequent contact results in tissue injury or a disease state. In certain circumstances previous exposure is unnecessary, and the same effects can result from primary exposure. Note that this reaction may or may not actually have a defensive function.

The classification of the hypersensitivity states in use includes the four types of Gell and Coombs, to which a fifth type was added and, as a result of recent better understanding of some other conditions, later a sixth, miscellaneous, group.

It is important to realize that a given clinical state— asthma, anaphylaxis, drug reaction—may be the expression of more than one type of hypersensitivity reaction, and that more than one type can contribute to a disease in the same patient (see later).

Classification (Gell and Coombs with two added groups) Table 7.1

Type I—anaphylactic type or immediate type
Occurs in hay fever, extrinsic asthma, drug reactions.
Type II—cytotoxic type
Occurs in transfusion reactions, haemolytic disease of the newborn, autoimmune diseases of blood elements.
Type III—immune-complex-mediated type
Examples are: serum sickness, glomerulonephritis, vasculitis— erythema nodosum, erythema induratum, polyarteritis nodosa.
Type IV—delayed-hypersensitivity type
e.g. contact dermatitis, caseation necrosis in Tb.
Type V—stimulatory type
as in thyrotoxicosis.
Type VI—miscellaneous group
e.g. gram-negative endotoxic shock, haemorrhagic shock syndrome of dengue fever, hypocomplementaemic membranoproliferative glomerulonephritis.

Type I—anaphylactic type or immediate type
Atopic individuals, who make up about 10% of the population, have a familial hereditary predisposition to anaphylactic allergy which often presents in infancy

or childhood with eczema, hay fever, asthma, or allergic rhinitis. These patients often develop multiple allergies to antigens encountered daily or seasonally in the environment, such as house-dust mites, pollens, animal dander, spores from mouldy hay.

In atopics or non-atopics who develop anaphylactic reactions of Type I there is either a solitary tissue or organ involved or systemic involvement of multiple organs as in generalized shock.

A significant proportion of atopics are reported to have a deficiency of IgA in their serum and mucous membranes in childhood which is corrected at a later age but which indirectly influences the development of the atopic state. Lack of secretory IgA ('the antiseptic paint of the mucous membranes') allows allergens to enter the mucosa and trigger an IgE antibody response leading to an immediate local hypersensitivity reaction. It is known that IgE antibody response is regulated by various different T cell subpopulations.

Some workers have suggested alternatively that response in these patients may be due to lack of suppressor effect by suppressor T cells, which would promote an IgE antibody response, but these suggestions have not been fully proved so far.

Mechanism of anaphylaxis (Fig 7.1)

Anaphylaxis is normally mediated by IgE antibodies which bind to the surface membranes of basophils and mast cells by their Fc regions. Mast cells are predominantly perivascular and present in abundance in the respiratory tree, g-i tract (omentum and mesenteries), and skin. This distribution, incidentally, corresponds to the tissue distribution of IgE-forming cells, which predominate in respiratory and g-i mucosa.

Table 7.1
Comparison of different types of hypersensitivity

	Type I Anaphylactic	Type II Cytotoxic
Common clinical conditions	allergic rhinitis, hay fever, extrinsic asthma, drug reactions, eczema	transfusion reaction, haemolytic disease of newborn (Rh), Goodpasture's synd., autoimmune + drug-induced haemolytic anaemias, thrombo-cytopenia
Antigen	usually exogenous pollen, mites from house dust, drugs	cell surface of RBC, basement membrane
Mediators	IgE—on mast cells, basophils, IgG	IgG, M, A ± complement system
Medium of passive transfer to normal subject	serum antibody	serum antibody
Skin test with antigen (intradermal)		
Appearance	wheal, flare	—
Maximum reaction	30 min	—
Histology	vasodilatation, oedema, eosinophilia, degranulated mast cells	immunofluorescent staining shows linear deposition of antibody and complement factors on basement membrane

Type III Immune complex	Type IV Delayed type	Type V Stimulatory
localized—extrinsic allergic alveolitis, erythema nodosum, extrinsic asthma *systemic*—rheumatoid arthritis, glomerulonephritis, polyarteritis nodosa	caseation reactions, transplantation rejection, contact dermatitis, insect bites	thyrotoxicosis
extracellular, fungal, parasitic, bacterial, viral	cellular or extracellular	cell surface
IgG, M, A ± complement system	Killer T cells, macrophages, lysomal enzymes, and lymphokines	IgG (called long-acting thyroid stimulant)
serum antibody	lymphoid cells transfer factor	serum antibody
erythema + oedema	erythema + induration	—
3–8 h	24–48 h	—
acute inflammatory reaction with polymorph infiltration and thrombosis in cases of vasculitis + deposited immune complexes	perivascular infiltration, first with polymorphs, then with mononuclears	—

Fig 7.1 Mechanism of Type I (anaphylactic)

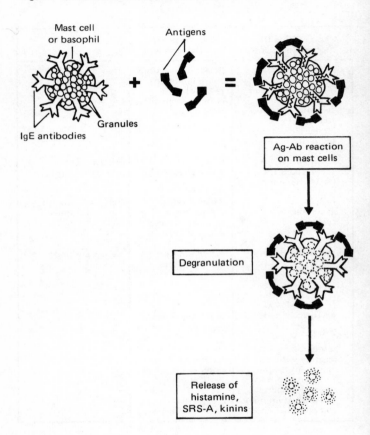

and their regional lymph nodes, with very few being found in spleen or subcutaneous lymph nodes. Mast cells are the tissue counterpart of the basophils, which are a rich source of histamine in blood.

There is no difference between the number of IgE molecules per basophil (10 000–40 000) in atopic and non-atopic individuals.

Reaction between allergen molecules and cell-bound IgE (so bridging the free receptors of the latter) activates the enzymatic sequences which lead to de-granulation of the basophils and mast cells and release of chemical mediators such as histamine, SRS-A (slow-reacting substances of anaphylaxis), prostaglandins, and kinins, which cause vasodilatation, increased capillary permeability, smooth muscle contraction, and attraction of eosinophils, at the site of reaction. The clinical manifestations of allergic rhinitis, hay fever, extrinsic asthma, anaphylactic drug reactions, or insect bites, can all be related to the biological activities of the vasoactive amines released by this mechanism. Eosinophilia often accompanies these conditions. Eosinophils also collect in tissues where the immediate hypersensitivity occurs in order to phagocytose the immune complexes and release their eosinophil granular contents which neutralize the his-tamine and other vasoactive amines released by the mast cells.

Diagnosis

A large number of the commoner antigens have been commercially purified for skin testing or inhalation provocation tests to identify the offending antigen, and for subsequent desensitization. Antihistamines must be stopped at least 3 days before such tests. A positive skin test results in a wheal and flare within 30 minutes, subsiding in 2-3 hours; a positive inhalation provocation test precipitates the asthmatic symptoms, usually quite mildly *but adrenaline should always be at hand in case severe anaphylaxis occurs.*

A large array of more sophisticated tests is also available to detect IgE antibody against a particular allergen, such as radio-immunoelectrophoresis and the radio-allergoabsorbent test. The basophil degranulation test has also been used, with variable results.

Treatment

Antihistamines, bronchodilators, and sodium cromoglycate (SCG) are the commonly used symptomatic treatments, in addition to advising avoidance, as far as is possible, of the allergen. They are useful for mild cases and in children, some of whom grow out of their sensitivity as they approach puberty, but it should be noted that the bronchoconstriction of asthma is thought to be caused mainly by SRS-A, which is unaffected by antihistamines—hence their ineffectiveness in this condition.

In severe cases specific desensitization should be considered. Desensitization therapy involves giving a course of subcutaneous injections of the relevent allergen, starting with a low dose and gradually increasing successive doses. The success of such therapy depends on accurate identification of the allergen and selection of appropriate desensitizing doses. The results of different series, and with different allergens, have varied, from 60% to 83% symptomatic relief being claimed in some. The improvement is believed to be due to development of IgG blocking antibodies in response to the repeated injections; these may bind the allergen on entry, before it can react with the IgE antibodies.

Recently IgG antibody which binds to mast cells and basophils has been described, but it is much less effective at causing degranulation of the cells. The exact contribution of antibody is ill understood, but it could explain the response of asthma to steroids, which is otherwise difficult to explain.

Type II—cytotoxic type
Mechanism (Fig 7.2)

Cytotoxic immunity is mediated by antibodies of IgG, IgM, or IgA class directed against cellular or membrane antigens such as red cells or transplant cells, or basement membrane respectively. The complement system is involved whenever activated.

When an antigenic cell reacts with IgG (combining at the F_{ab} region), opsonization is promoted by the existence of the surface receptors on polymorphs and macrophages for the (free) F_c region of the IgG. Similarly, when the complement system is activated by IgG and IgM antibodies reacting with cells, the C_{3b} receptors on the phagocytes promote immune adherence and further phagocytosis, as already mentioned in Chapter two.

When the antigen-antibody reaction occurs on basement membrane instead of on cell membrane, as in Goodpasture's syndrome (glomerulonephritis and haemorrhagic pneumonitis due to circulating anti-basement-membrane antibody), the complement activation causes an inflammatory reaction and polymorph infiltration, releasing proteolytic enzymes which damage the basement membrane. When the complement

7.10

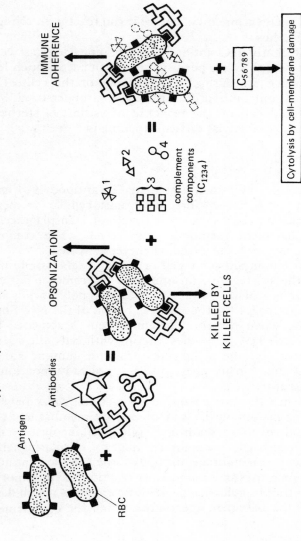

Fig 7.2 Mechanism of Type II (cytotoxic)

activation reaches the stage of C_8 and C_9, the resulting phospholipase activity damages the basement membrane *and* cell membrane and causes cell lysis.

While nucleated cells may be able to repair cell-membrane damage, non-nucleated cells such as red cells are unable to do so and are inevitably lysed.

Diseases involved
These fall into three main groups:
- blood group incompatibilities
  transfusion reactions—ABO
       —minor groups
  haemolytic disease of the newborn
     —Rh incompatibility
     —ABO incompatibility;
- autoimmune diseases—haemolytic anaemias
      —thrombocytopenias
      —Goodpasture's syndrome;
- organ transplants. If a transplant survives the delayed (Type IV) hypersensitivity reaction of the host, antibody response against histoincompatible antigens of *vascular endothelium* of the transplant may occur with the same sequence as in *Fig 7.2*. When this happens, platelet adherence in the donor-tissue blood vessels precipitates thrombosis of the vessels and ischaemic necrosis of the donor organ.

Transfusion reactions
Mismatched transfusions involving the major blood groups are potentially fatal. The natural isoagglutinins anti-A and anti-B are IgM antibodies which are highly efficient at activating complement and producing instant intravascular haemolysis. When this occurs on a major scale it can cause haemoglobinuria and renal shutdown. The isoagglutinins fortunately cannot cross the placenta to harm the fetal blood cells.

Haemolytic disease of the newborn (HDN)
Incompatibility between mother and child is the commonest reason for HDN. In the temperate western countries Rh incompatibility is the major cause, since about 15% of their populations are Rh-negative, but paediatric experience shows ABO incompatibility to be a commoner cause in tropical African countries.

HDN due to ABO incompatibility
ABO incompatibility in the newborn is caused by IgG antibodies (which, unlike IgM, can cross the placenta) against A or B fetal cells. Not only may such haemolytic antibodies be present before the first pregnancy, and therefore affect the first child, but it is also quite unpredictable whether there will be trouble in later pregnancies. What induces these antibodies in the mother is not known: it is believed they may arise in response to one or more of the multitude of infections encountered in the tropical environment which may cross-react with blood-group antigens. Such antibodies are reported to be more common in tropical countries.

ABO incompatibility is generally milder than Rh incompatibility and kernicterus is uncommon, but exchange transfusions are nevertheless often needed.

The diagnosis of ABO incompatibility in the newborn is often a problem, since the direct Coombs test is usually negative, and the indirect test cannot be used. The direct test is negative because a baby's red cells have only a few antigen sites to react with maternal antibody which gains entry to the fetal circulation. The amount of antibody on the cells is usually thus insufficient to allow agglutination of red cells by the antihuman globulin (AHG) used in the test (see below). The indirect test will not work on maternal serum, on the other hand, because the natural maternal IgM isoagglutinins interfere with the demonstration of IgG haemolysins unless tedious separation is carried out first.

Rh incompatibility

Rh incompatibility occurs in about 1/250 live births in those populations with a 15% Rh-negative prevalence. Small quantities of fetal cells leak into the maternal circulation from the second trimester onwards, but these do not excite a detectable anti-D response in the mother, suggesting that the important immunizing event is a major leak at the time of placental separation. About 17% of mothers carrying an ABO-compatible Rh-incompatible fetus become immunized during their first full-term delivery. If there is also ABO incompatibility the incidence of Rh immunization is about ten times less, as the ABO isoagglutinins destroy the leaking cells before their Rh antigens can immunize the mother. There is also an individual variation in maternal response to Rh+ fetal cells; about one-third of mothers who are Rh– fail to respond to any quantity of Rh+ cells.

Once a mother is immunized, however, any subsequent pregnancy with an Rh+ fetus is likely to lead to HDN with severity increasing with each successive pregnancy.

The harmful anti-Rh antibodies in HDN are IgG-7S which, as just mentioned, can cross the placental barrier and cause fetal complications. Very often these antibodies are not demonstrable on saline agglutination and require the use of antihuman globulin (AHG) for demonstration. In this case they are called 'incomplete antibodies' but in fact there is nothing odd about the antibodies themselves, the difficulty lies in the site of the Rh antigen.

Cell membranes are not smooth surfaces like a billiard ball, but folded and crenated, and while some antigens are right on the surface, others, such as the Rh, are situated at the bottom of a fold. When an antibody is able to easily attach by one of its Fab regions to one red cell and by the other to another one, agglutination occurs easily in saline (*Fig 7.3a*). When one Fab region has to stretch deeply into the membrane to reach the antigen (*Fig 7.3b*), however, the other Fab region cannot reach antigen on another red cell, and agglutination will not occur unless AHG is added to bridge the free Fc regions and link the RBC. This is what is meant when we speak of incomplete antibodies; in fact the antibodies are normal, it is the process of agglutination which is not complete without the help of AHG, owing to the site of the antigen.

One of the greatest successes of applied immunology has been the suppression of Rh immunization by giving Rh antibody i.m. or i.v. to all Rh- mothers within 24 hours of labour, abortion, or accidental placental haemorrhage during the first gestation prior to Rh immunization. With the right dose and timing 99% of maternal immunization can be prevented and the safety of the next Rh+ fetus assured. This prophylactic procedure has to be carried out in every pregnancy. The 1% failure rate may be explained on the basis of inadequate dosage of· antibody, or of pre-existing maternal immunization, because once active immunization has begun in the mother the passive administration of antibody is useless.

The usual dose of purified anti-D serum is 100-300 µg i.m. or 100 µg i.v. In the case of major (over 10 ml) transplacental haemorrhage the dose is 25 µg i.m. for every ml of fetal blood estimated to be in the maternal circulation.

Similar immunotherapy is difficult even to try in ABO haemolytic disease of the newborn because we

Fig 7.3 Diagrams of agglutination reactions

7.3a Saline agglutination

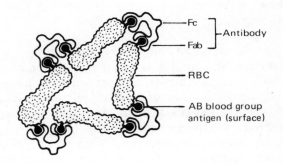

Fc ⎫
Fab ⎭ Antibody

RBC

AB blood group antigen (surface)

7.3b Direct Coombs test

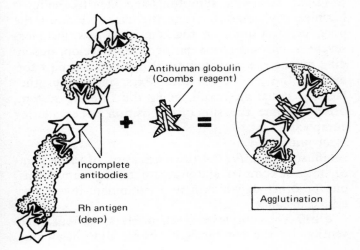

Antihuman globulin (Coombs reagent)

Incomplete antibodies

Rh antigen (deep)

Agglutination

are completely ignorant of how and when the maternal antibodies arise.

Autoimmune haemolytic diseases

The mechanism of cell damage and destruction in these is similar to that just outlined for blood-group incompatibilities (see also p 9.7).

Type III—immune complex-mediated type

An immune complex is an antigen-antibody complex which may activate or interact with complement, depending on the class of antibody involved and the size of the complexes present. Immune complexes are formed in various parts of the body and circulate under various circumstances such as infections, neoplasia, connective-tissue diseases, autoimmune diseases, drug reactions, and serum sickness. In about 98% of instances, the immune complexes may cause transient, reversible symptoms and then be rendered harmless by removal from the circulation by the phagocytic system. In the remaining few instances severe or chronic tissue damage may develop, depending on the site and amount of immune-complex formation, the size of the complexes, and many other factors. Renal glomeruli, being the filtering system, often become the site of deposition of circulating complexes.

Mechanism

As illustrated in *Fig 7.4* the mechanism of tissue damage may be complex and intricate, taking many forms, one or other of which may predominate in any particular instance.

● Immune complexes by themselves, without intervention by the complement system and phagocytes,

Fig 7.4 Mechanism of Type III (immune complex)

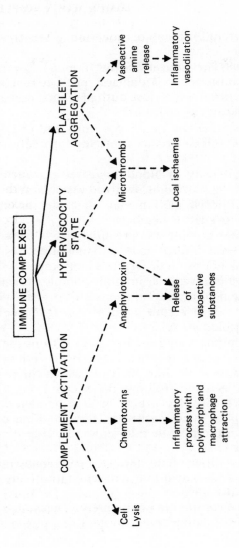

may cause mild basement-membrane damage and proteinuria;

● complement activation by immune complexes causes vasodilatation, fluid and protein exudation, and phagocytic infiltration; all of these perpetuate tissue damage;

● in the processes of phagocytosis and cell death, phagocytes release tissue-damaging proteolytic enzymes;

● hyperviscosity of blood, increased platelet adherence and sluggish blood flow from vasodilatation, and perivascular inflammation may all cause thrombosis and so produce tissue necrosis;

● immune complexes precipitated in vessel or bronchial walls induce acute inflammation, resulting in erythema nodosum or farmer's lung respectively;

● massive intravascular immune-complex formation and complement activation may result in anaphylactic shock in cases of serum sickness, e.g. from repeated use of heterologous ATS.

In both primary and secondary infections the time lag between appearance of antibody in response to antigen results in various phases in which the proportions of antigen and antibody differ (*Fig 7.5 a, b*). All these phases can play a part in development of immune-complex hypersensitivity, though some of the effects produced may be transient and self-healing.

Antigen phase I
During the initial phase antigen may sequestrate in the tissue spaces, where it may have no effects until free antibody diffuses there in phase III and reacts with it to form immune complexes. These may activate complement at the site and start an inflam-

Fig 7.5 Antigen-antibody proportions in infections

7.5a In a primary immune response

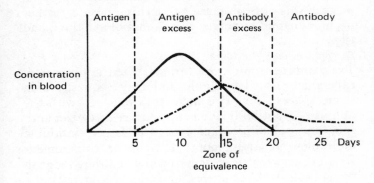

7.5b In a secondary immune response

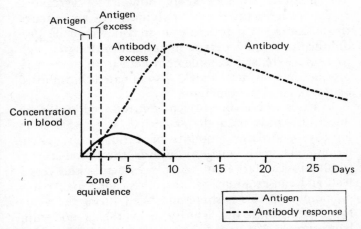

Note: In both primary and secondary immune responses the antigen or soluble antigen-antibody complexes can sequestrate harmlessly in tissue spaces or vessel walls. In subsequent phases of the response, however, free diffusing antibody can reach such sites and react with the deposits there, thus activating complement and causing inflammatory damage.

matory process and consequent tissue damage. This is believed to be one of the possible immunopathological mechanisms of glomerulonephritis, besides other haemodynamic factors such as renal blood flow, and filtration rate.

Antigen excess phase II

The immune complexes formed when antigen is in excess are usually soluble and may sequestrate in tissue spaces; their size increases, however, with the number of antibody molecules attached to the antigen, and solubility decreases. The larger, insoluble molecules are thus more efficient in complement fixation, and hence more harmful when they lodge in vessel walls or tissue spaces.

Zone of equivalence and antibody excess Phase III

The immune complexes are now large aggregates, easily phagocytosed by polymorphs, and hence tissue damage by proteolytic enzymes may be predominant. If they persist in circulation long enough to cause extensive complement activation, they may produce anaphylactic shock, disseminated thrombosis, or Raynaud's phenomenon.

In cases where the antigen is introduced locally by injection, or is naturally localized in a tissue as in leprosy, and large amounts of antibody are circulating, release of antigen towards the blood-stream results in formation of complexes across the vessel wall and causes an intense vasculitis called the Arthus phenomenon, this is sometimes seen during the treatment of lepromatous leprosy as erythema nodosum leprosum (ENL).

A similar mechanism operates in farmer's lung, which is due to the inhalation of actinomycetes spores.

Table 7.2
Clinical manifestations of immune-complex diseases

Generalized diseases	Components of immune complexes
1) Rheumatoid arthritis	IgG-anti-IgG (anti-IgG is the rheumatoid factor which usually belongs to IgM class) + complement components
2) Systemic lupus erythematosus	DNA-anti-DNA + complement components
3) Nephropathies (glomerulonephritis + nephrotic syndrome)	Streptococcal antigen and its antibody ⎤ Malarial antigen and its antibody ⎥ + complement components Hepatitis B antigen and its antibody ⎥ ? antigen + immunoglobulin ⎦ *this forms the major group of cases*
4) Polyarteritis nodosa	Some cases—hepatitis B antigen + antibody + complement
5) Serum sickness with ATS or penicillin	The serum used + its antibody + complement system
Localized diseases	
1) Farmer's lung	Thermophilic actinomyces spores + antibody
2) Erythema nodosum	*M tuberculosis* antigens + antibody (45% of cases) Other bacterial or drug antigens + antibody
3) Erythema leprosum	*M leprae* antigens + antibody + complement
4) Penicillin Arthus type reaction	Benzylpenicillin bound to body protein to form antigen + its antibody

These lodge in the bronchial tree and first cause an immediate hypersensitivity state, manifest as an acute attack of asthma; later a further attack occurs (after 6–12 hours) when immune complexes localize at the site and initiate an inflammatory response with oedema and bronchial constriction. This is a good example of the coexistence of two types of hyper-sensitivity response—Type I and Type III—and treatment has to be designed accordingly.

The search for immune complexes in immune-complex diseases is carried out on blood and in tissues. The common methods used on blood are the precipitation test with C_1, ultracentrifugation, electron-microscopy, and complement consumption assay; there are many other tests, however, and new ones are being discovered and published all the time. The commonest methods of detection of immune-complex deposits in tissues are by immunofluorescence and electronmicroscopy. Trying to detect the offending antigen is often a tedious and unsuccessful task, though streptococcal, malarial, hepatitis B, and DNA antigens have all been detected (Table 7.2).

Treatment

Steroids are anti-inflammatory—by stabilizing the lysosomal membranes of phagocytes they prevent release of inflammatory vasoactive and proteolytic enzymes. Antihistamines and sodium cromoglycate may be helpful in those conditions precipitated and localized by a Type I reaction, such as farmer's lung. Antihistamines also counteract the vasoactive amines released by complement activation. Immunosuppressive drugs such as azothiaprine and cyclophosphamide have also been used in some of these states.

Type IV—delayed hypersensitivity

This is mediated by T cells, and its mechanisms in contact dermatitis, transplant rejection, and caseating necrosis have been adequately covered in Chapter three on cell-mediated immunity. The major factors causing tissue damage in delayed hypersensitivity are the proteolytic enzymes released from the lysosomes of activated macrophages. Lymphotoxin and killer T cells have a variable contribution depending on the host tissue susceptibility.

Type V—stimulatory

In thyrotoxicosis an IgG (non-complement-fixing) antibody has been discovered which reacts with the same thyroid receptors as thyroid-stimulating hormone (TSH) and stimulates the thyroid to secrete thyroxine for a longer period than does TSH; hence it has been named long-acting thyroid stimulator (LATS). Recently some additional antibodies have been defined and implicated in the aetiology of thyrotoxicosis which are human-specific, unlike LATS which is assayed in mice.

Miscellaneous group

Recently at least three disease states have been described which are caused by activation of the alternate pathway of the complement system. These are:
  a) gram-negative endotoxic shock
  b) dengue fever haemorrhagic shock (some cases)
  c) hypocomplementaemic mebmbranoproliferative glomerulonephritis.

As mentioned in Chapter two, the biologico-pathological results of complement-system activation can be identical whichever activation pathway is involved.

The above classification clarifies the different types of hypersensitivity states and the immunopathological mechanisms involved in them. One has, however, to be cautious in attributing any particular clinical syndrome, such as a drug allergy or bronchial asthma, to any one type without an adequate history and laboratory, skin, and provocation tests. The allergic states caused by common drugs like penicillin or aspirin may fall into any of the four main types, or combinations of them, as mentioned above in the case of extrinsic asthma in which Type 1 hypersensitivity occurs first and then localizes the Type III immune complexes by inciting an inflammatory response.

The other point worth noting is that in Tb or leprosy, in which the CMI response is defensive, there is also an intense antibody response which complexes with the mycobacterial antigens released during treatment to precipitate the Type III hypersensitivity reactions. Thus, while caseation necrosis is attributed to delayed hypersensitivity, ENI is due to immune-complex vasculitis.

Chapter eight

IMMUNOLOGICAL TOLERANCE

Immunological tolerance is defined as antigen-specific immunological unresponsiveness. When an organism encounters an antigen, it either responds to it by producing humoral antibody or sensitized T cells, and memory cells, or it develops immunological tolerance to the antigen in question. In the first case a second contact with the same antigen within a few weeks or months results in an enhanced secondary response, in the latter case in no immune response. If the second contact occurs after a very long period, however, even in a previously tolerant organism, a positive immune response may now occur, due to the presence of fresh non-tolerant immunocompetent cells newly formed from stem cells.

Immunological tolerance must be distinguished from immunological suppression: tolerance is antigen-specific, while suppression is a generalized depression of immunological response to all antigens and is induced by certain drugs, irradiation, or disease. For tolerance to be induced, the organism must at some stage in its life be exposed to the antigen.

The normal immune response involves first of all recognition of the antigen by specific lymphocyte surface receptors; these then react by blast transformation, cellular proliferation, and differentiation, to serve the two functions of the system: the effector mechanisms, and memory. The effector mechanisms, the antibodies and sensitized cells, then act specifically on the antigen.

The mechanisms involved in immunological tolerance are many and intricate (see *Fig 8.1*). It may be of the *central type*, which results from interference with either the recognition phase or the cellular phase of induction of immunity, or it may be of the *peripheral type*, due to any blocking process which prevents existing effector mechanisms neutralizing or attacking an antigen.

Our aim in hypersensitivity states, autoimmune diseases, and organ and transplant rejection is to produce immunological tolerance to specific antigens; in the case of cancer, however, our object is to reverse the tolerance which has developed, and to achieve immunostimulation, in order to encourage rejection and killing of the neoplastic tissue. The greatest immunotherapeutic success so far has been in the prevention of Rh-negative mothers from being sensitized by their Rh-positive babies by giving them anti-Rh antibodies at the times when fetal cells are leaking significantly into the maternal circulation.

Fig 8.1 Consequences of antigen exposure to specific immune components

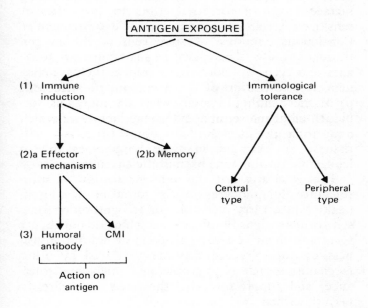

Central immunological tolerance
Clonal elimination
This form of tolerance depends on complete absence of production in the body of lymphocytes with antigen-specific receptors for an antigen or tissue; it is one of the explanations why we do not normally reject some of our own native tissues—autotolerance.

There is good evidence that if an antigen is present at the time when the haemopoietic stem cell is differentiating to become an immunocompetent lymphocyte, it prevents the formation of lymphocytes bearing surface receptors for itself; thus no antibodies or sensitized T cells are formed against it subsequently. Continuous exposure of stem cells to the antigen throughout life is necessary to maintain such tolerance and even so, under circumstances such as malignant transformation of the haemopoietic stem cells or of the lymphoid system, what are known as 'forbidden clones' of lymphocytes may be formed which may then produce autoantibodies to attack self-tissues; for example, in some lymphomas and in leukaemia autoimmune haemolytic anaemia occurs.

This is clearly not the only mechanism of auto-tolerance: lymphocytes may be found in the body in health which carry receptors for recognition of some self-tissues such as fibroblasts yet which do not appear to attack them *in vivo*. This form of nonresponsiveness or autotolerance may be produced by other mechanisms such as split tolerance, high-zone tolerance, and suppressor cells; the latter have already been described.

Low-zone (split) and high-zone tolerance

For every antigen and animal there is a range of antigen dose described as optimal because the animal responds to it with an immune response. If a lower (suboptimal) dose of a soluble antigen is repeatedly injected into the body of such an animal (the continuous but limited secretion of thyroxine into the circulation *in vivo* represents such a situation), the result (provided it is a first encounter with the antigen) is the development of *'low-zone'* or *'split' tolerance.* Thereafter, subsequent challenge with what would normally be an optimal dose of the tolerated antigen for such an animal fails to elicit any immune response, indicating that repeated exposure to low doses of the antigen has specifically inactivated some of the lymphocytes which bear its specific receptors.

In fact in this type of tolerance it is the T cells specific for the antigen which have become tolerant, while the antigen-specific B cells have not, but as the B cells cannot function and produce antibodies without T helper cells, the over-all effect is tolerance. Low-zone tolerance of this type is easily reversed, however, by infections or trauma serving to modify the antigen slightly, whereupon the body is able to recruit T helper cells which, with the already sensitive B cells, can now form antibodies to the antigen in question. A good example of this is the development of thyroid autoantibodies following viral thyroiditis.

Note that low-zone tolerance can only be artificially induced in an individual who has not previously been primed or sensitized by the antigen concerned, and who therefore has no memory cells for it. Once an individual has been primed by exposure to an antigen at its optimal dosage and has developed memory cells, only high-zone tolerance can thereafter be effectively induced against that particular antigen. Note also that persistence of the antigen is necessary for the maintenance of low-zone tolerance, or a new generation of T cells will arise which are not tolerant.

High-zone tolerance is induced by exposure of an animal to supraoptimal doses of an antigen, whereupon both T and B cells, although originally sensitive, now become tolerant to the antigen concerned. A good example of such an antigen is immunoglobulin.

Again persistence of the antigen is necessary for maintenance of high-zone tolerance, as fresh immuno-competent T and B cells are continuously being formed from stem cells and these have all the time to be rendered tolerant.

Suppressor cells
There is fairly good evidence that there is a set of lymphocytes in the body, mainly belonging to the T cell pool, which regulates immune response by supres-sive action on both the humoral and CMI responses. They are antigen-specific and may act directly on T and B cells, or through a secretory molecule which acts by macrophage intervention. In this way suppres-sor T cells appear to be responsible for maintenance of autotolerance.

Some animal work suggests these suppressor cells become fewer in number with ageing of an organism; this would explain the finding of increased circulating autoantibodies in the elderly even in health.

Suppressor cells inhibiting transplant rejection have been reported in some patients with prolonged sur-vival of transplanted organs.

Peripheral immunological tolerance
Blocking soluble antigen
When a parasite or tumour secretes large quantities of antigen into the circulation, the antibodies or cells formed against it are neutralized in the circulation

before they can reach the target site. This results in an ineffective immune response. The same phenomenon occurs with tissue antigens, which are released continuously into the blood-stream during tissue cell membrane turnover.

Enhancing and blocking antibodies

Enhancing antibodies are antibodies 'against' a tissue, which in practice protect it by covering up the antigenic site at which it would normally be attacked by T killer cells. Both the enhancing antibodies and the killer cells are formed against a common surface antigen; the antibody is usually non-complement-fixing and harmless to the tissue concerned. Such antibodies have been reported in progressive cancer patients and in some patients with long-surviving transplants.

Blocking antibodies typically appear in patients treated for Type I hypersensitivity by desensitization. The blocking antibody (IgG or IgA) has a strong affinity for the antigen and mops it up before it can reach and combine with cytotropic IgE antibodies.

Blocking soluble immune complexes

Soluble immune complexes (antigen/antibody, Ag/Ab, complexes) are often formed when there is excess antigen circulating in the body, and they may continue to circulate for a long time. Such complexes can bind directly to circulating T or B cells carrying the specific antigenic receptor for the antigen concerned, without triggering them; they can interfere with all forms of killer cell activity specific for that antigen in the body; and recently it has come to be believed that they may also trigger suppressor cell activity on behalf of the antigens concerned.

Soluble immune complexes thus depress the immune system at various levels, including blocking immune recognition and induction as well as interfering with killer cells. One or all of these mechanisms may be involved in the success which has been achieved in preventing maternal Rh isoimmunization.

The mechanisms described are the most important of those involved in producing immunological tolerance, but not the only ones; many other factors, such as the physical state of the antigen (monomeric or polymeric), the age of the patient, and drugs being given, play a part and need to be considered when attempting to induce tolerance in a patient therapeutically. As a result, the effects of immunological manipulations are not always predictable, nor always those desired.

It should also be noted that more than one mechanism may be involved in autotolerance to any body constituent, thus helping to ensure that autotolerance is maintained even if one mechanism fails.

Chapter nine

AUTOIMMUNE DISEASE

Autoimmune diseases (AID) are diseases resulting from immunological destruction of the body's own tissues following disruption of autotolerance. Ideally, to be absolutely certain that autoimmunity is the cause of a disease, all possible extrinsic infective causes should have been excluded; this has not in fact been done for all the diseases mentioned in this chapter although they are all currently accepted as of autoimmune aetiology.

All autoimmune diseases share certain common factors

• the tendency to develop autoantibodies to specific organs clusters in families. Similarly the tendency to develop non-organ-specific antibodies and non-organ-specific autoimmune diseases (e.g. antibodies against connective tissue, and rheumatoid arthritis) also runs in families, but the two types rarely occur in the same families. Thyroid diseases, for example,

often coexist in a family or in patients with pernicious anaemia, but connective tissue disease is unlikely to be found in
the same family or the same patients. Moreover, gastric parietal
cell antibodies are present in over a third of patients with autoimmune thyroid disease even without, in the majority, any
clinical manifestations of pernicious anaemia; similarly antinuclear factor is present in about half of patients with rheumatoid arthritis (RA) without any clinical evidence of systemic
lupus erythematosus (SLE) in most of them

- most AID are commoner in females
- hypergammaglobulinaemia is regularly present in AID
- presence of autoantibodies against different body constituents is a constant feature of AID and a useful diagnostic
criterion, although their presence in themselves is not enough
to make a diagnosis of AID. Many acute infections, such as
viral hepatitis, stimulate production of antinuclear antibody
and anti-smooth-muscle antibody for a short period; these
transient autoantibodies are usually entirely IgM class, however, while those of AID are predominantly IgG class
- the course of AID is variable and not always progressive.

Classification of AID (Table 9.1)

Some AID can be neatly classified as organ-specific
conditions, and others as non-organ-specific, but
there remain many others which fall into an inter-
mediate category, having features of both types.

The organ-specific AID are, as already mentioned,
characterized by the presence of autoantibodies
specific for the organ involved, as in thyrotoxicosis.
In non-organ-specific AID, on the other hand, the
autoantibodies are directed against a general body
constituent such as nucleoprotein, connective tissue,
or an IgG immunoglobulin, but not against any
antigen specific to the organs affected by the disease.
Other differences between the two polar types of

Table 9.1

Organ-specific	Intermediate	Non-organ-specific
1. Thyroid diseases —thyrotoxicosis —Hashimoto's thyroiditis —primary myxoedema	1. Myasthenia gravis	1. Systemic lupus erythematosus
	2. Pemphigus vulgaris	2. Discoid lupus erythematosus
	3. Bullous pemphigoid	3. Scleroderma
2. Autoimmune atrophic gastritis and pernicious anaemia	4. Phacogenic uveitis and sympathetic ophthalmia	4. Dermatomyositis
	5. Ulcerative colitis Crohn's disease	5. Mixed connective tissue diseases
3. Primary autoimmune Addison's disease	6. Goodpasture's syndrome	6. Rheumatoid arthritis
4. Blood disorders —autoimmune haemolytic anaemia thrombocytopenia leucopenia	7. Primary biliary cirrhosis	
	8. Chronic active hepatitis Cryptogenic cirrhosis	
5. Some few cases of male infertility	9. Sjögren's disease	
6. Some few cases of premature menopause		

Table 9.2

Organ-specific AID	Non-organ-specific AID
Familial tendency, with clinical and serological overlap within the groups, e.g. Hashimoto's patients often have parietal cell antibodies, with or without pernicious anaemia and vice versa. Clinically, 15% of pernicious anaemia patients have thyroid diseases and 55% have thyroid antibodies	Serological and clinical overlap also occurs within families; e.g. one-third of systemic lupus erythematosus (SLE) patients have rheumatoid factor. SLE and rheumatoid arthritis may also be found in different members of the same family
Organ damage is often related to intense round-cell infiltration of the organ	The damage is related to immune-complex deposition in the tissues
In health autotolerance of the organs involved is maintained by low-zone (split) tolerance; this can easily be terminated in experimental animals to reproduce the disease picture and study its various aspects	Well-established tolerance in health to the antigens concerned makes it difficult to reproduce the disease experimentally
Natural animal models exist, e.g. the obese chicken for myxoedema	Natural animal models such as NZB mice and SLE dogs are the only way of studying the disease experimentally
Treatment consists of replacement of hormones in those cases affecting endocrine glands or (in pernicious anaemia) Vit. B_{12}	Treatment has to be by immunosuppressive therapy and anti-inflammatory drugs

AID are given in Table 9.2

Autoantibodies are, as we have said, useful diagnostic markers of AID, but they may also have other significance in some of the diseases, as shown in Table 9.3.

The autoantibody is not always actually involved in the causation of the disease, e.g. the mitochondrial

Table 9.3

Disease	Autoantibodies present against	Medical significance
Hashimoto's thyroiditis Primary myxoedema	Thyroid microsomes Thyroglobulin Cell surface	Present in 98% of cases. Their presence excludes colloid goitre and a psychiatric cause for patient's symptoms
Thyrotoxicosis	Thyroglobulin Thyroid microsomes Cell surface (LATS) (LATS protector)	High levels indicate co-existent Hashimoto's thyroiditis and contra-indicate surgery or irradiation treatment High levels are associated with pretibial oedema which may respond to steroid therapy
Pernicious anaemia	Parietal cell Intrinsic factor	Useful to differentiate PA from other megaloblastic anaemias, and subacute combined degeneration of the cord from other spinal cord diseases
Primary Addison's disease	Adrenal cells	Excludes Tb adrenalitis

[continued overleaf

Table 9.3 continued

Disease	Autoantibodies present against	Medical significance
Myasthenia gravis	Skeletal muscle or Myoid cells of thymus	Striated muscle antibody indicates a thymoma is present (possibly in an ectopic site if it is not in the anterior mediastinum)
Autoimmune (lupoid) chronic active hepatitis and cryptogenic cirrhosis	Nuclear antigens Smooth muscle Mitochondrial antibody	Allows differentiation from other forms of chronic hepatitis and cirrhosis
Primary biliary cirrhosis (PBC)	Mitochondrial antibody	Useful in differentiation from obstructive jaundice
SLE	DNA Other nucleoproteins	Severity of disease closely parallels anti-DNA antibody titres
Rheumatoid arthritis	IgG	High titres indicate worse prognosis

antibody found in primary biliary cirrhosis. Those antibodies which do have a causative relationship are further briefly discussed below.

Organ-specific diseases
• *Thyrotoxicosis* Long-acting thyroid stimulator (LATS) and LATS protector antibodies are IgG antibodies which, when they bind to the thyroid acinar cells, stimulate them to synthesize and secrete thyroid hormone. This can cross the placenta in pregnancy and produce a transient neonatal thyrotoxicosis. The

LATS protector antibodies are the human-specific antibodies mentioned on p 7.23.

● *Hashimoto's disease* Cytotoxic antibody against thyroid cell membrane is detectable in this condition and may be relevant to the disease.

● *Autoimmune haemolytic anaemia* may be subdivided into two types, the *warm antibody type* and the *cold antibody type*. The warm antibody type usually has IgG antibodies directed against red cell rhesus antigens; the cold antibody type may be subdivided further into cold haemagglutinin disease (CHD) and paroxysmal cold haemoglobinuria (PCH). CHD has IgM antibodies or cryoglobulins, usually directed against the I antigen system of the red cells while in PCH the autoantibody is an IgG directed against red cell antigen P (ref. p 7.9 and *Fig 7.2*).

● *Atrophic gastritis and pernicious anaemia* Parietal cell antibody may be related to the chronic inflammatory destruction of gastric mucosa seen in atrophic gastritis. This leads to marked reduction in secretion of intrinsic factor and acid. Vitamin B_{12} binding and absorption is further hampered by the additional presence of antibody to intrinsic factor in the gastric secretions which neutralizes what little intrinsic factor is secreted.

● *Primary infertility in males* Autoimmune orchitis is the cause of 3% of primary cases of male infertility; sperm-agglutinating antibodies may be partly responsible for it.

Intermediate group
● *Myasthenia gravis* The striated muscle antibody binds to the thymic myoid cells, setting up a thymitis

which causes release of a neuromuscular-blocking agent from the thymus which is believed to be responsible for the clinical features of the disease. A thymoma may stimulate pressure-induced thymitis and lead to the same result.

● *Goodpasture's syndrome*   This haemorrhagic pneumonitis and glomerulonephritis results from basement- membrane antibodies which bind to the basement membranes of alveoli and glomeruli and cause inflammatory damage. Passive transfer of serum from an affected patient into a monkey will reproduce the disease picture.

Non-specific group

● *Rheumatoid arthritis (RA)* The majority of adult rheumatoid patients have IgM rheumatoid factor in their serum, which gives a positive result with the routine laboratory (Rose-Waaler and latex) tests; these patients are known as seropositive patients. Nearly all juvenile cases, however, have IgG rheumatoid factor which does not react positively with the routine tests, and these patients are called seronegative; when they grow up they tend to remain seronegative.

The inflammatory joint damage in RA is related to formation of immune complexes between IgG and IgM rheumatoid factor in seropositive cases, and IgG and IgG rheumatoid factor in the seronegative cases. In both cases activation of the complement system takes place with release of proteolytic enzymes from phagocytes, causing the tissue damage.

● *SLE* The skin, renal, and CNS involvement in this disease is related to tissue damage caused by the

Fig 9.1 Diagram of sequence of formation of LE cells in vitro

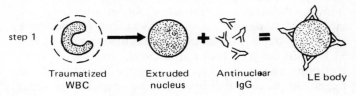

step 1

Traumatized WBC → Extruded nucleus + Antinuclear IgG = LE body

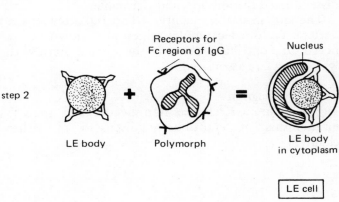

step 2

LE body + Polymorph = LE body in cytoplasm

Receptors for Fc region of IgG

Nucleus

LE cell

deposition of DNA-anti-DNA immune complexes at these respective sites. In some patients a lymphotoxin has been isolated which explains the finding of lymphopenia; warm antibody-type autoimmune haemlytic anaemia may also occur in the disease. The LE cell phenomenon described in SLE and some chronic liver diseases is related to the presence of antinuclear antibody in the sera of such patients. The mechanism involved in the formation of LE cells is shown in *Fig 9.1*.

● *Mixed cryoglobulinaemia* Cryoglobulins are usually circulating complexes formed between anti-immunoglobulin and immunoglobulin and they pre-cipitate deposits in various sites at low temperature; they may occur in a variety of conditions such as RA, SLE, lymphomas, leukaemia. Such circulating cryo-globulins can cause hyperviscosity of the blood and hence hypercoagulability, ending up in vasculitis, disseminated thrombosis, and ischaemia.

The autoantibodies mentioned are but a few of the better-established examples which are known or be-lieved to contribute towards the disease state with which they are associated.

Summary diagram
Fig 9.2 summarizes the non-specific and specific mechanisms of cytotoxicity discussed in earlier chapters.

Fig 9.2 Summary diagram: Mechanisms of target cell destruction

NON-SPECIFIC MECHANISMS	SPECIFIC IMMUNE MECHANISMS	

NON-SPECIFIC MECHANISMS

1. Phagocytosis by polymorphs and macrophages.

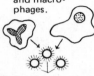

2. Proteolytic enzymes released during phagocytosis (1) can be cytotoxic; can also directly activate some complement factors

3. Activation of alternate pathway of C system activation can enhance (1) and (2) by opsonization. Final activation of C_8 and C_9 causes membrane damage and cell lysis.

4. Other cytolytic humoral agents in the body such as gastric acid, lysozymes and basic polypeptides.

SPECIFIC IMMUNE MECHANISMS

Antibody-mediated

a) Opsonic antibodies promote phagocytosis and intracellular killing

b) Immune complexes activating complement enhance opsonization and direct lysis too

c) IgG antibody promotes cell killing through non-T, non-B lymphoid killer cell

(*Note:* macrophages, polymorphs, and non-T, non-B lymphoid killer cells possess surface receptors for IgG antibodies.)

Cell-mediated

a) T killer cells

b) Activated macrophages show enhanced phagocytosis and intracellular killing*

c) Lysosomal release extracellularly is cytotoxic to bystander cells

d) Armed macrophages show antigen specific target cell cytotoxicity

e) Lymphotoxin can be cytotoxic too

* Activated macrophages do not show antigenic specificity, they show increased bacteriolysis and virolysis to bystanders as well as the triggering antigen.

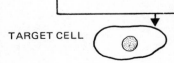

TARGET CELL — A pathogen, host tissue cell, transplanted cell, or neoplastic cell.

Chapter ten

IMMUNODEFICIENCY DISEASES

Immunodeficiency is a self-explanatory term including both disorders of the specific and nonspecific immune responses of the body, the former mediated by lymphocytes, the latter by phagocytes and complement.

It is an extensive subject to cover briefly, and this chapter will first discuss the immunodeficiency diseases (IDD) classified according to the nature of the immune defect, then the diagnostic tests available, and lastly treatment as far as it is understood at present.

Classification
The classification 'tree' (*Fig 10.1*) may be recognized from Chapter three where it appeared in simpler form, in connection with transfer factor therapy for acquired cell-mediated immune deficiencies, not further

Fig 10.1

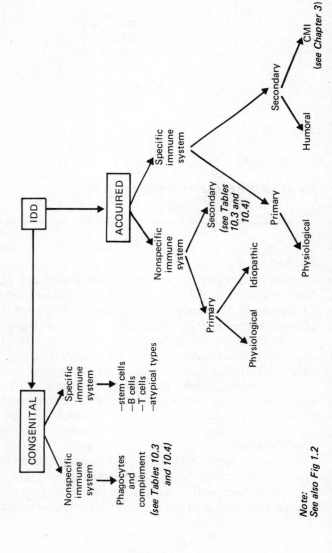

Note:
See also Fig 1.2

discussed here. *Congenital* immune deficiency is divided into defects of the lymphoid system and those
of the phagocyte and complement systems. *Acquired*
deficiency is divided into *primary*—physiological and
idiopathic (so far no known cause)—and *secondary*,
further divided into humoral and cellular deficiencies.

CONGENITAL IMMUNODEFICIENCY STATES

Lymphoid system (Table 10.1)
B cell defects (humoral antibody system)
B cell disorders usually appear 3–6 months after birth,
when the protective maternal IgG antibody disappears
and the infant, incapable of synthesizing his own antibodies, develops repeated pyogenic bacterial infections
of the g-i and respiratory tracts. Four types are listed
in Table 10.1, three due to B cell deficiency, one in
which B cells are present but antibody formation is
still defective. In this group the peripheral blood B
lymphocyte count may be normal.

T cell defects (CMI system)
The thymus is derived from the 3rd and 4th branchial
arches as an epithelial organ and subsequently populated by lymphoid stem cells coming from the haemopoietic tissues. Absence or anomalies of the thymus
are thus associated at times with anomalies of the
great vessels, heart, and thyroid and parathyroid
glands. Sometimes a rudimentary or normal thymus is
present in the neck, having failed to migrate normally
into the anterior mediastinum. Children with thymic
deficiency, and hence T cell deficiency, commonly

Table 10.1
Congenital ID states affecting
the lymphoid system and its function

B cell defects
Infantile X-linked agammaglobulinaemia (Bruton type)
Non-sex-linked agammaglobulinaemia
Selective immunoglobulin disorders (dysgammaglobulinaemia)
Agammaglobulinaemia with B cells present

T cell defects
Thymic and parathyroid aplasia (DiGeorge's syndrome)
Thymic hypoplasia + fibrous thyroid (Good's syndrome)

Stem cell defects
Autosomal recessive agammaglobulinaemia (Swiss type), SCID
X-linked thymic hypoplasia (Gitlin type)
Nezelof's syndrome
Reticular dysgenesis
Associated with short-limbed dwarfism
Associated with adenosine-deaminase (ADA) deficiency

Atypical states
Wiskott-Aldrich syndrome (X-linked recessive)
Ataxia telangiectasia (autosomal recessive)
Immune amnesia
Deficiency of certain lymphokines (e.g. MIF secretion cannot be induced in some cases of chronic mucocutaneous candidiasis)

present with viral, fungal, or protozoal infections (see Chapter three, p 3.10). The two common types are given in Table 10.1.

Stem cell defects—severe combined immunodeficiency disease (SCID)
Stem cell defects affect, of course, both cell systems; not only does the thymus fail to become populated by lymphoid cells but the humoral system is also de-

fective. The thymus shadow on Xray is usually absent or reduced, and there is marked lymphopenia. Other haemopoietic elements may also be affected, and other congenital abnormalities are often present.

Seven examples are listed in the Table; while these may appear unfamiliar and rare conditions, it has been estimated from European studies that stem cell defects may be one of the commonest genetic immune defects and contribute up to 10% of infant mortality from that cause after 3 months of age.

Atypical states

This group includes conditions which do not fit well into the first three categories. Four syndromes are listed in Table 10.1.

In the Wiskott-Aldrich syndrome there are defects in cellular immunity and low levels of IgM and sometimes IgG, reflecting diminished ability to recognize and react to certain carbohydrate antigens. Children with this defect have raised levels of IgA, and present with thrombocytopenia, eczema, and recurrent infections.

In ataxia telangiectasia there are low levels of IgA and sometimes IgG, and diminished T-cell immunity, with cutaneous and cerebral telangiectasia. Affected children suffer from increasing cerebellar ataxia and recurrent pulmonary infections.

Phagocytes and complement system

Phagocytosis was considered at some length in the first three chapters. It is an important non-specific defence mechanism involving the polymorphs, monocytes, and fixed macrophages of the reticuloendothelial system. Various cellular and serum factors are together intimately involved in the full process of phagocytosis, in which at least four distinct stages can

be defined:
- *chemotaxis*—migration of motile phagocytes towards the focus of infection;
- *adherence and opsonization*—adherence between the target or antigen and the phagocyte cell membrane is essential for opsonization to follow;
- *ingestion*;
- *intracellular killing*.

Chemotaxis
Chemotaxis is initiated by the generation of chemotactic factors by:

a) some organic products (especially from non-pathogenic organisms);

b) pathogen + antibody + activated complement system resulting in C_{3a} and C_{5a}, $\overline{C_{567}}$ which are chemotactic;

c) some pathogens also produce the three chemotactic factors just mentioned by alternate pathway activation;

d) some pathogenic proteinases activate C_3 and C_5 directly;

e) dead tissue-cell constituents.

Adherence and opsonization
Inert particles, some non-pathogens, and a few pathogens adhere readily to phagocyte cell membranes and are easily ingested, but many pathogens do not. The phagocytes, however, possess surface receptors for the F_c region of IgG and for C_{3b}, and once such pathogens have reacted with IgG antibodies or the C_{3b} component of activated complement, they then also adhere readily to the phagocytes. The possible mechanisms of adherence and opsonization are:

a) nonpathogens and inert particles adhere spontaneously

b) pathogen + IgG antibody

c) pathogen + antibody (IgG or IgM) + $\overline{C_{1423}} \rightarrow C_{3b}$

d) pathogen or its product + complement activation by alternate pathway C_{3b}, which promotes immune adherence and phagocytosis.

Ingestion

Once the pathogen adheres to the cell membrane of a phagocyte, the phagocyte throws out pseudopodia to enclose it within a vacuole which results from fusion of the plasma membrane round the pathogen. This is termed the phagosome.

Intracellular killing

Once a phagosome containing an organism is within the phagocyte cytoplasm, the process of intracellular killing starts. The phagosome fuses with the cyto-

Table 10.2
Bactericidal mechanisms of
cytoplasmic granules of phagocytes

Cationic protein (phagocytin) bacteriostatic and bactericidal activity by interaction with the anionic groups on bacterial membrane

Hydrolytic enzymes (lysosymes)—bacteriolysis by direct action on cell walls, especially of gram-positive bacteria

H_2O_2 is bactericidal in the high concentrations in which it is present particularly in polymorphs

H_2O_2 + **myeloperoxidase** + **a halide (usually Cl)**—the two latter oxidizable co-factors greatly potentiate the bactericidal activity of H_2O_2. Various bacterial species and fungi are inhibited or destroyed by this mechanism

Acid pH is bactericidal for some organisms

plasmic granules, which discharge their contents into it, digesting and destroying the target organism by the variety of proteolytic enzymes they consist of. Cytoplasmic granules containing acid hydrolases, as in macrophages, are called lysosomes. Table 10.2 lists the proteins and other bactericidal agents of the cytoplasmic granules of macrophages and polymorphs.

The characteristic defects and other clinical or pathological findings associated with defective phagocytosis are summarized in Tables 10.3 and 10.4. For convenience congenital and acquired conditions are considered together. By 'quantitative defect' is meant a deficiency in the number of phagocytes in general, as occurs in some of the congenital conditions listed in Table 10.3 and also in acquired granulocytopenia from drug or chemical (e.g. benzene and derivatives) hypersensitivity. By 'qualitative defect' is meant a defect in one of the four stages of phagocytosis listed above. Defects in the complement system (Table 10.4) are of course, as just mentioned, closely involved in chemotaxis and opsonization.

ACQUIRED STATES

Primary
A physiological hypogammaglobulinaemia usually occurs in infants below 3–5 months of age (but sometimes later, even up to a year) when maternal antibody is disappearing and their own antibodies have not yet formed.

A group of patients also exists with prolonged hypogammaglobulinaemia of IgG, IgM, IgA, in whom no cause is known—idiopathic hypogammaglobulin-aemia.

Secondary

Some of the acquired immunodeficiency states involving cell-mediated immunity have been briefly and partly covered in Chapter three (p 3.18). Other circumstances under which *CMI* may become deficient are as follows:

malnutrition

• children with kwashiorkor fail to achieve Mantoux conversion after BCG vaccination and the same children develop a rather severe form of measles when they contract the disease; this suggests depression of CMI. Atrophy of the thymus and of lymphoid tissue has also been reported in kwashiorkor. Intracellular bacterial killing in phagocytes is reduced though normal opsonization and phagocytosis take place. Serum levels of complement components are also subnormal;

infections

• non-specific transient loss of CMI also occurs in certain infections such as measles, syphilis, and leprosy. In some viral diseases, such as measles and infectious mononucleosis, the virus actually infects and multiplies within the lymphoid cells which may be a reason for depression; in other conditions circulating immune complexes could be responsible for depression of lymphocyte reactivity;

malignancies

• CMI may be depressed in advanced malignancies, this is seen particularly in Hodgkin's disease;

irradiation, cytotoxic drugs, and corticosteroids

• depending on dose and the chemical constitution of each agent, lymphocyte reactivity can be variably depressed by these agents.

Table 10.3
Disorders of phagocytes

Disorder	Defect in phagocytosis	Comments
A. Congenital		
1. Congenital chronic neutropenia	Quantitative	
2. Cyclic neutropenia	Quantitative	Every 3 weeks
3. Lazy leucocyte syndrome	Quantitative and chemotaxis	Severe neutropenia because of impaired marrow release
4. Chediak-Higashi syndrome	Chemotaxis and intracellular killing and neutropenia	Autosomal recessive inheritance; polys have giant granules with less proteolytic enzymes
5. Schwann-Diamond syndrome	Ingestion Quantitative	Associated pancreatic insufficiency and low IgM and low IgA
6. Congenital ichthyosis	chemotaxis	
7. Myeloperoxidase deficiency	Chemotaxis and intracellular killing	Associated with candidiasis
8. Chronic granulomatous disease (CGD)	Intracellular killing	Commonest type is sex linked abnormality
9. Job's disease (like CGD)	Intracellular killing	Only in males, associated with pigmented skin, red hair and enzyme defect
10. Congenital splenic defect	Quantitative defect of macrophages which leads to low opsonic capacity	Hypoplasia or aplasia
11. Serum inhibitor of leukocyte mobility	Chemotaxis	Lack of natural antagonist to inhibitor of chemotaxis

Disorder	Defect in phagocytosis	Comments
B. Physiological		
12. Physiological abnormality in newborn	Chemotaxis, opsonization, intracellular killing	
C. Acquired		
13. Neonatal neutropenia	Quantitative	Associated with maternal agglutinins to fetal antigens
14. Sickle cell disease leading to hyposplenism	Opsonization and quantitative defect of macrophages	Associated with Salmonella and pneumococcal infection
15. Diabetes mellitus	Chemotaxis, opsonization and ingestion in ketoacidosis	Insulin addition corrects chemotaxis
16. Acquired neutropenia	Quantitative defect	Drug or other chemical hypersensitivity
17. Acute myeloid leukaemia	Quantitative defect	Defect in maturation
18. Chronic myeloid leukaemia	Intracellular killing	

Table 10.4
Deficiency of complement factors or related enzymes

Deficiency	Functional defect	Comments
A. Congenital		
1. Apparent *C_{1q} deficiency	None	Associated with Swiss hypogammaglobulin-aemia
2. *C_{1r} deficiency	Repeated infections and renal and skin disease	Lethal
3. C_2 deficiency	Some healthy and some show disease	Renal, skin, and haema-tological disorders
4. C_3 deficiency	Repeated bacterial infections	Lethal
5. C_4 deficiency	SLE-like disease	
6. C_5 deficiency	Opsonic defect	Recurrent bacterial infections
7. C_6 deficiency	None	Healthy
8. C_7 deficiency	None	Healthy
9. C_3 hypercatabolism	Defective chemo-taxis, opsonization, leading to recurrent infections	Deficiency of a natural inhibitor of C_{3b}
B. Physiological		
10. Newborn have lower levels of C_3, C_5 and properdin factors	Defective chemo-taxis, opsonization	Prone to infection
C. Acquired		
11. Hypocomplemen-taemia *C_1 subcomponents	Opsonization	Deficient synthesis in cirrhosis and kwashi-orkor

The acquired states affecting *humoral immunity* are:

agammaglobulinaemia with thymoma (spindle-cell tumour)

● there is a deficiency of all immunoglobulins and antibody responses which may be associated with eosinopenia and/or red cell aplasia; the mechanism involved is not known;

low IgG due to

● excessive loss as in lymphangiectasis, enteropathies, the nephrotic syndrome;

● increased rate of catabolism as in myotonia atrophica (Steinert's disease) or from drug treatment (e.g. steroid therapy);

low IgA and IgM (with normal IgG)

● secondary to lymphoreticular malignancies;

● in toxic dysgammaglobulinaemia occurring in uraemia, cytotoxic therapy, coeliac disease, diabetes.

Generally speaking in these conditions IgM is the first immunoglobulin to fall, followed by IgA, and IgG is the last, to be affected.

Clinical features of both congenital and acquired deficiency states of the lymphoid system

Some ID states cause neonatal infections; in others the common childhood infections—measles, chickenpox, mumps—are severe or fatal; in others complications of vaccination develop when live attenuated vaccines are given. Recurrent infections are common, and respond to treatment slowly.

Infections may be:

● *bacterial*—recurrent upper and lower respiratory infections are frequent, sometimes associated with meningitis;

● *viral*—the common childhood viral infections such as

measles and chickenpox take an unusually severe, often fatal course;

- *mycotic*—candidiasis and cryptococcosis are common;
- *parasitic*—pulmonary infections with *Pneumocystis carinii*, malabsorption due to *Giardia lamblia* infections, and heavy and generalized strongyloidiasis are seen.

With a few excptions, such as chronic granulomatous disease (CGD, Table 10.3), *lymphadenopathy and/or splenomegaly are absent in infections in the immunodeficiency syndromes*—a useful clinical guide.

Other features

- G-i disorders, e.g. chronic diarrhoea, coeliac disease;
- recurrent skin eruptions, e.g. chronic eczema or morbilliform eruptions;
- impaired weight gain and growth (largely preventable by rearing in a germ-free environment);
- autoimmune manifestations, e.g. haemolytic anaemia and thrombocytopenia, and rheumatoid arthritis;
- malignancies, e.g. lymphoreticular neoplasia and leukaemia, are common;
- associated congenital abnormalities, e.g. hypoparathyroidism (causing tetany) and hypothyroidism;
- disseminated vaccination reactions when live attenuated vaccines such as BCG, smallpox, polio, measles, rubella, mumps, are used.

Do not give live attenuated vaccines in the presence of immunodeficiency

INVESTIGATION FOR
IMMUNODEFICIENCY STATES

One may wish to investigate for deficient
- humoral immunity
- cell-mediated immunity
- non-specific immune factors.

Humoral immunity

The following tests are used:

- *differential white count* to detect lymphopenia or neutropenia. A normal count, however, is compatible with some ID states;
- *serum protein electrophoresis*, though this only reveals gross albumin and globulin abnormalities;
- *immunoelectrophoresis*, carried out with both polyvalent antiserum and with monospecific antisera for IgG, IgM, IgA, etc; the control should be a normal sample matched for the age of the patient;
- *radial immunodiffusion quantification* (Mancini). Wells are made in agar containing a monospecific antiserum against IgG, IgM, or IgA, as shown in *Fig 10.2*. Five of them are filled with standard WHO reference serum, at 100%, 50%, 25%, 10%, and 5% strengths; the remaining three wells are then filled with the sera under investigation. Precipitation rings form round the wells by reaction with the antiserum incorporated in the agar, and the test serum concentrations are read off from a graph.

The same technique can be used for the estimation of some complement factors; although these are normally present only in small amounts, the technique is sensitive, when low concentrations of antiserum are used in the agar, down to about 10/μg/ml.

As the finding of a normal immunoglobulin concentration measured by these methods does not exclude

Fig 10.2 Radial immunodiffusion technique for quantitation of immunoglobulins

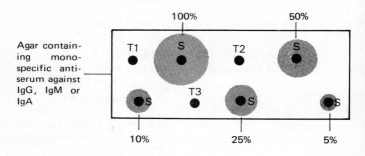

Agar containing mono-specific anti-serum against IgG, IgM or IgA

Key

S—standard WHO reference serum
T—test serum samples

antibody deficiency, it is essential also to test the response of these patients to antigenic stimulation.

Assessment of antibody formation
Two types of antibodies are sought:

● 'natural antibodies, e.g. isohaemagglutinins A and B, or heterophile antibodies against sheep or rabbit cells;

● active immunization antibodies, using DPT vaccine, pneumococcal or *H influenzae* polysaccharides, or Vi antigen and flagellin from salmonellae.

Recommended regimes of immunization and the techniques of detecting and quantitating antibody response can be found in the *WHO Bulletin* Report on primary immunodeficiencies.

Cell-mediated immunity
The thorough investigation of CMI is quite a task, and

the common tests employed for it are:
- differential white count, and peripheral film morphology;
- delayed-type skin reactions;
- *in vitro* stimulation of lymphocytes to divide and form blast cells;
- release of macrophage migration inhibition factor (MIF— Chapter three);
- skin graft rejection.

The *skin* and the *lymphocyte stimulation* tests can be used to investigate pre-existing immunity as well as to assess the capacity for active sensitization. The common antigens used for skin testing are mumps, trichophytin, PPD, candida, streptokinase, and streptodornase. Practical details are available in the WHO report.

For active immunization DNCB (2-4-dinitrochlorobenzene) is applied to the skin as a sensitizer (use 10% solution in infants). It binds to skin proteins to provoke T cell sensitization, and an erythematous induration results on challenge after 14–21 days.

Skin heterografts are occasionally performed, since graft survival is prolonged or indefinite (total nonrejection) in T cell deficiency in spite of the genetic incompatibility between donor and recipient.

In vitro *lymphocyte transformation tests*

PHA transformation Certain plant lectins (proteins) such as phytohaemoagglutinin (PHA) and concanavalin are called mitogens because they induce mitosis of lymphoid cells without previous sensitization. It is believed this happens because most T cells naturally possess receptors for PHA on their cell membranes and therefore undergo blast transformation on primary contact with them.

PPD or malarial antigen-induced transformation Since memory
T cells from a person previously exposed and sensitized to
agents such as mycobacteria and malaria parasites have membrane receptors for these antigens, blast transformation results
on contact with such antigens *in vitro*, as with mitogens, but
the number of responding cells is much less.

Mixed leucocyte culture reaction It has been observed that,
without any previous exposure, lymphocytes from one individual can recognize those of another allogeneic individual as
foreign because of the genetic disparity between their cell-
membrane antigens, and if cultured together both sets of cells
undergo blast transformation. To test the reactivity of the cells
from one person only, the other cell population is inactivated
with respect to its capacity to undergo blast transformation,
without affecting its viability and surface antigens. When the
two populations are mixed, only those of the test patient
undergo blast transformation (provided they are immunologically competent). In this test the proportion of cells under-
going transformation is less than in the PHA test but more
than in the PPD/malarial antigen test.

In all the above *in vitro* tests blast cells are recognized by direct microscopy and counting, and also
quantitated by the amount of radioactive tritiated
thymidine taken up for the synthesis of nucleoprotein
during blast transformation.

Both qualitative and quantitative T cell abnormalities may be recognized by these various tests, provided
reliable controls are used.

Macrophage migration inhibition factor

When sensitized lymphocytes are cultured with their specific
antigen—e.g. cells from a Mantoux-positive individual with
PPD—or if normal lymphocytes are cultured with PHA, macrophage migration inhibitory factor is released, which can be
shown to inhibit normal migration of macrophages as com-

Fig 10.3 Macrophage migration inhibition test

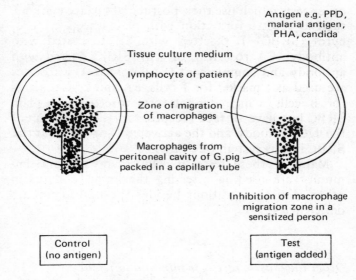

Antigen e.g. PPD, malarial antigen, PHA, candida

Tissue culture medium
+
lymphocyte of patient

Zone of migration
of macrophages

Macrophages from
peritoneal cavity of G.pig
packed in a capillary tube

Inhibition of macrophage
migration zone in a
sensitized person

Control
(no antigen)

Test
(antigen added)

pared with a control system.

Two plates are set up, as in *Fig 10.3*, one with and one without antigen (control). Guinea-pig peritoneal-cavity macrophages packed in a capillary tube are applied and, if the test cells are immunocompetent and react with the antigen, the zone of migration of the macrophages from the capillary tube in the test culture is much reduced compared with the control. Lack of immunocompetence, as in some IDD, results in normal migration of the macrophages, as in the control culture.

In some cases of chronic mucocutaneous candidiasis and SSPE (subacute sclerosing panencephalitis), for example, the patient's cells fail to produce MIF when cultured with candida and measles antigen respectively; sometimes this can be corrected by transfer therapy.

Differential T and B cell counts

For quantitation of T and B cells there are several other tests which use their postulated surface markers, such as rosette formation with plain sheep erythrocytes (SRBC)—E rosettes, with SRBC coated with antibody (EA rosettes), or with SRBC coated with antibody and complement (EAC rosettes). E rosettes are used as a marker for T cells, EA and EAC rosettes for B cells, which do not form rosettes with plain SRBC but have surface receptors for the Fc region of the IgG antibody and the activated C_3 which coat the SRBC in this system (see *Figs A.5, 6*).

Many of these tests of cellular and humoral immunity are used in assessing the immune status in other clinical conditions besides the basic immunodeficiencies.

Other diagnostic tests for immunodeficiency

Chest Xray A large thymic shadow in the anterior mediastinum is prominent at birth and in infancy; absence or hypoplasia can be seen on straight Xray or, with more precision, after inducing a pneumomediastinum. (Absence of an intrathoracic thymic shadow, however, does not prove absence of the thymus, as the latter may be ectopically situated, e.g. in the neck.)

Biopsy A somewhat risky procedure, and of limited value, is biopsy of lymph nodes, bone marrow, or rectal mucosa, after antigenic stimulation. The risk is infection, which commonly results if there is in fact immunodeficiency.

Tests of non-specific immunity
Complement system
There are two kinds of tests for the complement system: quantitative, using the radial immunodiffusion technique, and functional tests of the haemolytic capacity of the system. Although the two do often correlate, functional abnormality can occur without quantitative abnormality.

Phagocytosis
Quantitative abnormality of polymorphonuclear neutrophils is easily detected by a differential white count of blood, while macrophage function is assessed by a macrophage clearance function test with I^{125} PVP or carbon. Other tests done on polymorphonuclear neutrophils are the myeloperoxidase stain and candida-killing test. The nitroblue tetrazolium test (NBT) is especially useful in diagnosis of chronic granulomatous disease of childhood.

Multiple tests
It should be noted that in the investigation of immune status conclusions are never drawn from any single one of the tests described above. A battery of tests is carried out and deductions made from the over-all results.

TREATMENT

Lymphoid immunodeficiency is treated by one or more of the following procedures.

Replacement of antibodies
This has been carried out for B cell-deficient states such as Bruton's agammaglobulinaemia (see Table 10.1) using immunoglobulin preparations. This procedure is of no value, however, in the severe combined deficiencies (Swiss type).

Immunological reconstitution
a) Fetal thymic grafts are used to restore immunocompetence in T cell-deficient children, who usually possess competent stem cells which can mature to T cells in the presence of a fetal thymus. The graft is taken from a 12-week fetus, when the organ is still only epithelial and no problem of graft-versus-host reaction (see below) will arise, even when donor and recipient are not histocompatible.

Thymic extracts in the form of thymosin and other related substances have been used with some success in partial immunological reconstruction of T cell deficiencies. The E rosettes with SRBC increase, but usually the T helper effect in the IgG antibody response fails to be reconstituted by these extracts.

b) Bone marrow transplantation has been successful in many cases of SCID, provided the donor and recipient are histocompatible, and preferably also ABO-compatible; this usually implies a sibling donor.

The two major histocompatibility systems important to bone marrow transplant success are the serologically defined HLA antigens and the lymphocyte-defined antigens, the latter being investigated by mixed leucocyte culture.

In the event of incompatibilities being present, a fatal *graft-versus-host* (GVH) reaction is likely in an immunodeficient patient, as the transplanted cells are stem cells; these develop in the recipient into immuno-competent cells which immediately recognize the recipient's genetically different tissues as foreign and attack them.

A healthy person receiving an incompatible marrow transplant, of course, would reject the donor stem cells before they developed into immunocompetent cells, but this fails to happen in the immunodeficient recipient. In the GVH reaction the attack by the donor cells eventually results in liver, renal, and circulatory failure, and cachexia.

Transfer factor therapy

This has been partly dealt with in Chapter three, but is further mentioned here with reference to the treatment of other ID states. The greatest success of TF therapy has been in the Wiskott-Aldrich syndrome, but some cases of ataxia telangiectasia, chronic mucocutaneous candidiasis, and Swiss-type agammaglobulinaemia have responded favourably and acquired cellular immunity. Repeated injections are usually needed at regular intervals to maintain the immunity so acquired. A few cases with idiopathic acquired IgG hypogammaglobulinaemia have responded to transfer therapy, suggesting that their defect may be in helper T cells required for T-B cell co-operation in the IgG immune response (Chapter three).

Leucocyte transfusion

Recently attempts at immunological reconstitution in lepromatous leprosy by leucocyte transfusion have been reported, using infusion of donor whole-blood buffy coat; it appears to be unimportant whether the donor is lepromin-negative or positive. The preliminary reports are encouraging.

Technical appendix

This appendix deals mainly with a few essential immunological points relevant to common laboratory tests used in different fields of pathology, physiology, endocrinology, etc.

Common terms

Serum the fluid portion from clotted blood, i.e. plasma minus fibrinogen, prothrombin, factor V, and factor VII. To obtain serum blood is collected in a plain bottle and allowed to clot

Plasma the fluid portion of unclotted blood, with fibrinogen and other clotting factors except for divalent cations such as calcium. To obtain plasma blood is collected and mixed with an anticoagulant such as EDTA, heparin, sodium citrate, and the cells removed by sedimentation or centrifugation

Soluble reagent or solution a transparent clear fluid reagent

Suspension a translucent reagent (when well shaken) consisting of a particulate substance suspended in a fluid

Precipitation formation of visible complexes in a solution or in a clear semi-solid medium such as agar gel

Agglutination linking of smaller particles in a suspension to form larger coarse visible particulate complexes.

All immunological tests basically depend on the fact that all antibodies react with the antigen which stimulated their formation, and vice versa. For example the antibodies found in typhoid patients react specifically with salmonella organisms and their constituents, but not with shigellae or *Esch coli*.

It must be re-emphasized that most biological substances, such as bacterial or parasitic extracts or cells used in laboratory tests as an antigenic source or substrate, possess many antigens on their surfaces, some of these being of the same kind repeated on the surface, others being of a different kind and shape. For example a red cell from a group A individual has many A antigens on its surface, as well as Rh and minor blood group antigens. Such a cell, or any other substance possessing many antigens of one kind, is called a multivalent antigenic substrate.

Laboratory tests
Precipitation tests
The reagents used for precipitation tests are usually in solution when the test is to be carried out in the fluid state, but suspended antigenic substrate may be used if the test is being carried out in a semi-solid medium such as agar gel (*Fig 10.2*).

Principle

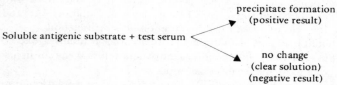

Soluble antigenic substrate + test serum

precipitate formation
(positive result)

no change
(clear solution)
(negative result)

All classes of antibody can give precipitation reactions as they possess two or more antigen-binding sites allowing them to bridge a multivalent antigenic substrate.

Precipitation usually occurs when the antigen-antibody ratio is optimal, or when there is anti*body* excess in the test system. Antigen-antibody complexes formed in anti*gen* excess are usually soluble, however, so in practice a titration is set up with a series of antigen dilutions to determine the best working range. This avoids the possibility of a false negative reaction from using an unduly strong antigenic substrate.

On the other hand, when the test is being used to detect an antigen in solution, the known antibody being used should be concentrated enough to detect the antigen if the latter is present in large amounts in the test solution. To avoid false negatives in this situation the test serum or solution should be set up in several serial dilutions.

Note
Antigen and antibody preparations, and test sera should be carefully stored to prevent loss of their biological activity, which should also be repeatedly checked. Microbial contamination of reagents or of a patient's serum can give false results.

Agglutination tests
Principle
Routine blood grouping is a common example of an agglutination test. Sample results with an unknown subject might be

Test RBC + anti-A serum	→	agglutination –
Test RBC + anti-B serum	→	agglutination –
Test serum + known group A RBC	→	agglutination +
Test serum + known group B RBC	→	agglutination +

(*Fig 7.3a*)

From these results it is apparent that this person is Group O and that he possesses the natural A and B isoagglutinins in his serum.

All classes of antibody may give agglutination reactions but IgM antibodies are the best agglutinins since they possess 5–10 antigen binding sites. The antigenic substrate, as in the precipitation test, should be multivalent for the reaction to occur.

One of the reagents, usually the antigenic substrate, is a suspension, e.g. of RBC or bacteria, but soluble antigens can be used if they are first linked to or reacted with RBC or latex particles. In the latex test for rheumatoid factor, for example, IgG immunoglobulins are linked to latex particles for use as the antigenic substrate.

Autoagglutination of the substrate can occur from faulty storage or contamination, so a suitable control with suspension alone has to be included in the test system to exclude false positive results. Test samples should also be taken and stored aseptically to prevent microbial contamination, which can also cause false positive results.

Both precipitation and agglutination tests can be done with

serial dilutions of the test samples to assess the titre of the reaction. If the test is then repeated on another sample from the same patient a week or ten days later, and a rising titre is observed, then active infection with the organisms concerned, or active disease in the case of an autoimmune disease, is confirmed.

Complement fixation tests (CFT)

The CFT is done on a patient's serum to detect the presence of complement-fixing antibodies (i.e. IgM and IgG) against soluble microbial or parasitic antigens, indicating previous contact with such agents. A rising antibody titre, as just mentioned, confirms the presence of active infection.

Principle
i) Known antigen + test serum + complement is incubated at 37°C for 30 min or longer.
ii) Sensitized sheep's red cells (i.e. coated with complement-fixing anti-SRBC antibodies) are added.

Results
i) No haemolysis in the second stage indicates that the serum did contain complement-fixing antibodies against the known antigen and reaction between these consumed the complement, leaving none to produce haemolysis in the second stage. This is a positive result, provided appropriate controls were set up to exclude other anticomplementary activity.
ii) Haemolysis means complement was not consumed in the first stage so there were no IgM or IgG antibodies in the test serum.

Controls
Appropriate controls are vital for reliable results in this test. An antigen control without test serum is necessary because

many microbial and tissue lipoprotein antigens can activate the complement system directly by the alternate pathway in the absence of any antibody to them in the test serum. A control with the test serum and no antigen is also needed because the test serum may contain soluble immune complexes formed *in vivo*, aggregated immunoglobulins, or microbial contaminants which may all activate the complement system by the classical or alternate pathways in the absence of an antigen. Finally a complement control is set up to ensure the potency of the source of complement used, and an SRBC control to exclude the possibility of old or deteriorating SRBC giving a false negative result by spontaneous haemolysis.

Immunofluorescence
Principle
This technique uses antibodies or antigens labelled with fluorescent dyes to recognize an antigen-antibody reaction in tissues, cells, or on cell surfaces; fluorescent dyes such as fluorescein isothiocyanate or rhodamine emit visible coloured fluorescence when excited by UV light.

Three main methods are used: the direct, the indirect, and the sandwich methods.

Direct immunofluorescence (Fig A.1)
This method is used to detect immunoglobulin molecules present on B cells. It is also used for detecting the immune complexes + activated complement factors which are deposited in diseased tissues in some disease states, e.g. the immune complexes in the glomeruli in glomerulonephritis and in the vessels in vasculitis of various kinds. The same method is also used to identify organisms in material cultured from patients.

The indirect test (Fig A.2)
This is used to detect autoantibodies against normal tissue

Fig A.1 Direct immunofluorescence

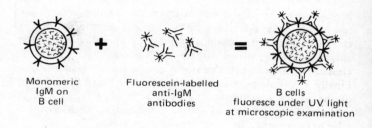

Monomeric IgM on B cell + Fluorescein-labelled anti-IgM antibodies = B cells fluoresce under UV light at microscopic examination

Fig A.2 Indirect immunofluorescence

step 1

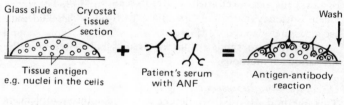

Glass slide — Cryostat tissue section

Tissue antigen e.g. nuclei in the cells + Patient's serum with ANF = Antigen-antibody reaction

Wash

step 2

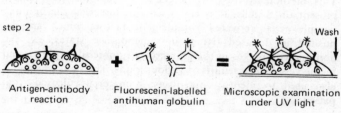

Antigen-antibody reaction + Fluorescein-labelled antihuman globulin = Microscopic examination under UV light

Wash

Fig A.3 Sandwich technique

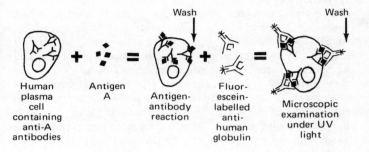

| Human plasma cell containing anti-A antibodies | Antigen A | Antigen-antibody reaction | Fluor-escein-labelled anti-human globulin | Microscopic examination under UV light |

antigens and antibodies against various microbes or parasites.
A tissue section used as antigenic substrate is reacted with the
patient's serum, and if antibodies are present they fix to the
tissue antigen and are detected by fluorescein-labelled anti-
immunoglobulin reagent as a second reaction. This second
reaction does not occur if there was no antibody present in the
test serum.

The sandwich test (Fig A.3)
This is essentially used to detect the number of plasma cells in
a lymphoid tissue which are secreting antibodies against a particular antigen. Known antigen is allowed to act on the lymphoid tissue concerned and if antibodies are present the
antigen-antibody reaction is detected by the later addition of
fluorescein-labelled antihuman globulin. Subsequent fluorescence in UV light indicates a positive reaction showing that
antibodies to the test antigen were present. (It is called the
sandwich test because the complex formed in a positive test
has 3 layers—antibody—antigen—antiglobulin—somewhat like a
sandwich.)

Radioimmunoassay
Principle
This method is highly sensitive and it can be used to detect substances present in the body fluids in minute quantities, such as hormones. The requirements are a supply of purified radiolabelled antigen of the kind it is desired to test for, and its specific antibody. Measured quantities of these two are then incubated together, alone (as a control) and with added test serum. If there is antigen present in the test serum it consumes some of the antibody, and less is available to react with the radiolabelled antigen. There is then more free radiolabelled antigen at the end of the test in the test sample than in the control sample.

Procedure (Fig A.4)
Two tests are set up for every sample.

i) Radiolabelled antigen + specific antibody.
ii) Radiolabelled antigen + specific antibody + test serum.

Fig A.4 Radioimmunoassay test

A.4a Radiolabelled antigen and antibody

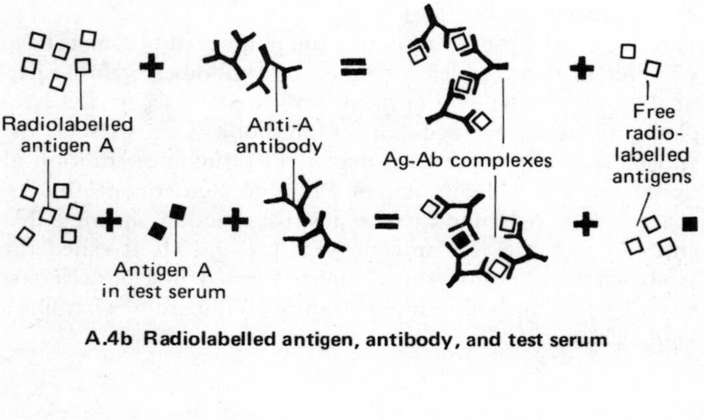

Radiolabelled antigen A   Anti-A antibody   Ag-Ab complexes   Free radio-labelled antigens

Antigen A in test serum

A.4b Radiolabelled antigen, antibody, and test serum

Results
If the residual free radiolabelled antigen in the two samples is equal, the test is negative and the test serum contained no antigen. If there is more free radiolabelled antigen in ii), the test is positive, and there was antigen present in the test serum.

Rosette tests
T cells
Human T cells possess surface receptors for SRBC and if T cells and SRBC are incubated together at 4°C the SRBC adhere to the T cell surface giving a rosette appearance under the microscope. These are known as E rosettes (E for erythrocyte).

Fig A.5   E rosettes

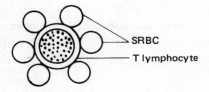

SRBC

T lymphocyte

B cells and macrophages
Human B cells and macrophages have surface receptors for the Fc region of IgG. If either SRBC coated with IgG-class anti-SRBC serum or chicken RBC coated with their corresponding antibody are incubated with B cells or macrophages at 37°C the coated RBC adhere and form rosettes as above. These are known as EA rosettes (E for erythrocyte, A for antibody).

If only B cells are to be detected the macrophages can be removed from the mixture by exposing them to carbonyl iron which they phagocytose; they are then removed by sedimenting them by magnetic force, the lymphoid cells remaining in the supernatant.

B cells can also be detected by the surface immunofluorescence test which detects the surface immunoglobulins which are their antigenic receptors, as mentioned above (*Fig A.1*).

Fig A.6 EA rosettes

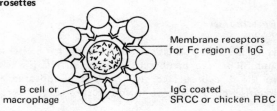

Membrane receptors for Fc region of IgG

B cell or macrophage

IgG coated SRCC or chicken RBC

For other immunological tests refer to Chapter ten, on immunodeficiency states and to Chapter two.

Suggested further reading

1. *Immunology for students of medicine.* J.J.H. Humphrey and R.G. White. Oxford, Blackwell Scientific Publications, 1970, 3rd edn.
2. *Essential Immunology.* Ivan Roitt. Oxford, Blackwell Scientific Publications, 1977, 3rd edn.
3. *T and B Lymphocytes.* M.F. Greaves, J.J.T. Owens and M.C. Raff. Amsterdam, Excerpta Medica; New York, American Elsevier Publishing Co., Inc., 1974.
4. *Clinical aspects of immunology.* P.G.H. Gell, R.R.A. Coombs, and P.J. Lachmann. Oxford, Blackwell Scientific Publications, 1975, 3rd edn.
5. *Progress in Immunology II.* Volumes 1–5. Leslie Brent and John Holborn (editors). Proceedings of the Second International Congress of Immunology, UK. Amsterdam, North Holland Publishing Co.; New York, American Elsevier Publishing Co., Inc., 1974.
6. *A Dictionary of Immunology.* W.J. Herbert and P.C. Wilkinson. Oxford, Blackwell Scientific Publications, 1976, 2nd edn.
7. *Cell-mediated immunity and resistance to infection.* WHO Technical Report Series No. 519, 1973.
8. *Immunology of parasitic infections.* Sydney Cohen and Elvio Sadun (editors). Oxford, Blackwell Scientific Publications, 1976.
9. *Developments in malaria immunology.* WHO Technical Report Series No. 579, 1975.
10. *Parasites in the immunised host.* Ciba Foundation Symposium No. 25. Amsterdam, Excerpta Medica; New York, American Elsevier Publishing Co., Inc., 1974.
11. *Prevention of Rh Sensitisation.* WHO Technical Report Series No. 468, 1971.
12. *Seminars in Haematology.* Vol. XI No. 3. Histocompatibility, immunosuppression and bone marrow transplantation. Jon J. van Rood (editor). New York, Grune & Stratton, 1974.
13. *Primary immunodeficiencies.* Report of a WHO Committee in Paediatrics. Vol. 47, No. 5, 1971.

Glossary of terms used in immunology

Note: the abbreviation *q.v.* is used sometimes in this glossary after a synonym. It stands for *quod vide* and means 'look under this alternative heading'.

Ab, ab abbreviation for antibody

Absorption a term used to refer to the use of reagents for removing antigens or antibodies from a mixture, necessary to purify antisera because the majority of antigens used in immunization procedures (e.g. in the laboratory) are highly impure and contain many unwanted antigen determinants which can induce antibodies which are likely to confuse the results of tests carried out on the resultant antiserum. The same method of absorption can be used to purify antigens (to remove the contaminants of antigenic preparations) if pure antisera are available

Acquired immunity = active immunity

Active immunity protection which develops as a result of an immune response to foreign substances or cancer cells

Adaptive immunity = active immunity

Adjuvant a substance such as aluminium hydroxide or complete Freund's adjuvant which nonspecifically enhances the immune response to the antigen it is used with. In the case of aluminium hydroxide the action is by strong adsorption of the soluble antigen onto its surface and subsequent slow release after injection into the tissues

Affinity the strength of firmness of binding between antigen and antibody

Ag, ag abbreviation for antigen

Agglutination clumping of *particulate* antigens, such as cells, bacteria, or latex particles by specific antibody which joins two cells by forming bridges between them

Agglutinin an antibody (or other substance such as a lectin) which causes agglutination of particulate antigens

AHG anti-human globulin; this contains antibodies directed against different components of human globulins, such as immunoglobulins, and some complement factors

Allergen an antigen which provokes an allergic or hypersensitivity reaction

Allergic response an altered host response, usually the result of previous contact with a substance, which produces a disease state or tissue damage

Allogeneic genetically dissimilar individuals within the same species

Allograft a graft derived from a genetically dissimilar individual of the same species

Anaphylactic shock a severe generalized shock syndrome caused by generalized release of vasoactive amines and other biological substances in the body. The clinical syndrome can be mediated by Type I, II, and III hypersensitivity states as well as by mechanisms which may activate the alternate pathway of the complement system in the body

Anaphylaxis the words anaphylaxis and anaphylactic reaction are also, confusingly, applied specifically to Type I or immediate-type hypersensitivity, although many of its clinical symptoms and signs also occur in other forms of hypersensitivity states

Anergy absence of CMI reaction or response to a delayed hypersensitivity test in a host after definite exposure to an antigen or disease, e.g. a negative lepromin test in lepromatous leprosy

ANF antinuclear factor antibody

Antibody an immunoglobulin capable of combining with a specific antigen through its antigen-binding sites

Anticomplementary a term referring to any reagents or test samples used in the complement fixation test (see Technical Appendix) which consume complement factors by activating the complement system on their own without the specific antigen-antibody reaction under investigation having taken place. These interfere with the complement fixation test commonly used for laboratory detection of antigens and antibodies

Antigen a substance which, when introduced into a host, elicits a specific immune response, humoral, cellular, or both.

Antigen-antibody complex = immune complex. A molecular complex formed of antigen and antibody molecules bound specifically together. They may be soluble or precipitating in type, depending on the number of antibody molecules in the complex

Antigenic combining site the site on the antibody molecule that combines specifically with the antigen

Antigenic determinant = antigen (see p 1.16)

Antigenic disguise an alteration in the antigenic constitution of an organism or cell which conceals its original identity

Antigenic drift a change or variation in the antigenic constitution of viruses with emergence of new strains

Antigenic variation modification and change of antigenic constitution of an organism during a certain infective episode which allows it to survive the host immune response

Antigenicity = immunogenicity. The potential of an antigen to stimulate an immune response in a particular host

Antiglobulin antiserum containing antibodies against different constituents of globulin protein

Antiglobulin test a test for detecting incomplete antibodies by use of antiglobulin reagent. In the *direct* test an antigen already coated with the incomplete antibody *in vivo* is sought; in the indirect test free soluble incomplete antibody in serum is reacted with the appropriate antigen in the laboratory in order to demonstrate it

Antiserum serum from an animal or human containing antibodies against a specified antigen

Antitoxin an antiserum containing antibody against exotoxin or endotoxin from a bacterium or fungus

Atopy a constitutional or hereditary tendency to Type I, anaphylactic immediate hypersensitivity

Attenuated vaccine a live preparation of micro-organisms which have been treated and cultured under special conditions leading to loss of virulence but retention of capacity to stimulate protective immunity

Autoantibody an antibody in a host capable of reacting with one of the host's own normal body constituents

Autograft transplantation of tissue from one site to another in one individual

Autoimmune disease a clinical disorder resulting from immunological destruction or manipulation of tissues or their products in the host, autoantibodies are commonly present in such cases, reflecting the immunological reaction to the autoantigens

Autologous derived from self

B cell B lymphocyte, bone marrow—or bursa—derived

BCG Bacille Calmette Guerin. A living attenuated bovine strain of *M tuberculosis* used as a vaccine to protect against human tuberculosis

Bence Jones protein Protein consisting of dimerized light chains which are secreted in the circulation, and appear in the urine, due to an unbalanced overproduction of light chains in monoclonal gammopathies and some other clinical states. The protein precipitates at 60°C in the urine and redissolves on further heating to 90°C

Blast cell a large, primitive-looking cell capable of division and differentiation

Blocking antibody an antibody that binds to an antigen and prevents it reacting similarly with another class of antibody or cell; often found in cases of Type I hypersensitivity after desensitization to the antigen

Blocking antigen a soluble exoantigen (an antigen released from an organism or cell) which reacts with an antibody or sensitized cells so that the latter are unable to react with the original source of the antigen, which may be a neoplastic growth or a parasite

Blocking immune complexes soluble immune (ag/ab) complexes with excess antigen sites available to react with and block antibodies and sensitized cells before they inflict damage on the original source of the antigen such as a parasite or tumour. The antibody molecule of the complex can also block killer cells (which act through their membrane receptors for the Fc region of IgG) before they damage the source of antigen

C complement.

C̄ activated complement

CFT complement fixation test

Carrier molecule a molecule which conjugates with a hapten *in vivo* or *in vitro* in order to render it immunogenic

Cell-mediated immunity (CMI) specific immunity mediated by sensitized T cells and their products

Central lymphoid organs the lymphoid organs essential for the embryological development of the functional lymphoid tissue necessary for immune response. The cellular events of proliferation and differentiation of lymphoid precursors in these organs are independent of antigenic stimulus

Challenge administration of a reagent a second or subsequent time to provoke an immunological reaction

Chemotaxis enhanced migration of cells towards a focus, caused by biochemical substances

Clonal selection theory the theory proposed by Burnet concerning antibody production, that a single antigen can only stimulate a reaction in a very small clone of lymphoid cells which carry surface receptors on them which enable them to recognize that determinant. The same clone cannot recognize another dissimilar antigen

Clone a family of cells derived by binary fission from a single parent cell, so that all the cells of a clone are genetically identical provided no mutation has taken place during the derivation process

Cold antibodies = cryoglobulin *q.v.*

Committed cell during the process of lymphocyte differentiation and maturation in the central or primary lymphoid organs a lymphocyte gains the capacity to recognize one specific antigen or a few very closely related molecules long before any question of antigenic stimulus arises; such a cell is described as being committed to that specific antigen. The progeny of such a cell or the antibody that may be secreted when it is stimulated maintain the same antigenic specificity and would not react with an unrelated antigen

Concomitant immunity = premunition; non-sterilizing immunity whereby partial resistance in a host to subsequent challenge with a parasite (or pathogen) is maintained by the presence of low-grade parasitaemia in the host

Coombs reagent antiglobulin reagent which has antibodies against the major serum immunoglobulins; some types also possess antibodies against components of activated $\overline{C_3}$

Coombs test = antiglobulin test $q.v.$

Delayed hypersensitivity a hypersensitivity state mediated by sensitized T cells and their products. It appears 24–48 hours after contact with the antigen, and can be transferred passively from a sensitized to a non-sensitized host by transfer of lymphocytes

DNC DNCB dinitrochlorbenzene; an organic chemical which is often used to assess immune competence of T cells in human subjects since it binds to skin protein and almost always sensitizes normal hosts

Eczema itching, inflammatory, non-contagious skin eruption, usually irregular in distribution and character, and showing redness, papules, vesicles and sometimes weeping

Electrophoresis a method of separating ionizable substances such as proteins or lipids by the virtue of their different rates of migration in an electric field between two electrodes

End cell a mature cell which is incapable of further division

Exchange transfusion replacement of a major part of the blood by simultaneously withdrawing it and replacing it with a transfusion of different blood

Fluorescein isothiocyanate a reactive yellow dye which combines with proteins in alkaline solution and emits intense green light when stimulated by ultraviolet light; often used to label antibody in immunofluorescence testing

Forbidden clones clones of lymphocytes which should not develop or survive in the body in health if autotolerance is to be maintained

Germinal centre a discrete nodular region, generally in secondary lymphoid organs, but sometimes in other tissues and in central lymphoid organs, consisting of an aggregation of lymphocytes, dendritic cells, and macrophages; related to development of humoral immunity in response to an antigenic stimulus. Germinal centre formation is dependent on T-B cell co-operation, which is also necessary for development of memory in B cell responses; it is also a site for localization of antigen in secondary lymphoid tissue

Glomerulonephritis a kidney disease primarily caused by injury and damage to the glomeruli

Granuloma a localized collection of macrophages, lymphocytes, fibroblasts and giant cells; some macrophages take on a characteristically altered appearance and are called 'epithelioid cells'

Gene a small functional unit of a chromosome, which controls a certain cell function by bearing the code for some part of a cell protein or enzyme

Gene product a product of a gene, in, on, or secreted outside the cell

Haemolysis lysis or rupture of red blood cells

Haemolytic anaemia anaemia caused by an increased rate of red cell destruction in the body

Hashimoto's disease chronic inflammatory damage to the thyroid, associated with focal round cell infiltration and formation of germinal centres

Hay fever acute nasal catarrh and conjunctivitis caused by a

Type I hypersensitivity reaction to pollen inhalation; sometimes associated with bronchial asthma as well

Histocompatibility antigens genetically determined isoantigens
on the membranes of nucleated cells which, if introduced
into another individual (i.e. transplanted) can provoke an
immune response and lead to graft rejection if the isoantigens
differ from the host's isoantigens. Some of these can be
recognized by the serological and cellular tests available so
far

Histocompatibility genes the genes controlling formation of
histocompatibility antigens

HLA human leucocyte locus A; the locus (site) on each of a
pair of chromosomes where the genes controlling the major
histocompatible antigens involved in transplantation work
are; these include the SD and LD antigens

Homograft = allograft *q.v.*

Heterograft = xenograft *q.v.*

Humoral antibody antibody present in body fluids such as
plasma, lymph, and (extracellular) tissue fluid

Humoral immunity immunity mediated by humoral antibodies

Hypergammaglobulinaemia raised serum gammaglobulin levels.
Immunoglobulins are the major components of the serum
gammaglobulins; rises in immunoglobulins (or antibody)
therefore cause rises in the serum globulins

Hyperimmunization a procedure whereby a host's immune system is optimally stimulated, often artificially, by an antigen

Hypersensitivity = allergy

Hypogammaglobulinaemia lowered serum globulin levels

Ig abbreviation for immunoglobulin

Immediate hypersensitivity = anaphylactic, Type I, hypersensitivity

Immune protected against a disease or diseases

Immune adherence a phenomenon whereby activated complement factor promotes the adherence of immune complexes
to phagocytes

Immune antibody antibody resulting from an active immune response as opposed to an isoantibody such as anti-A naturally present in some people and used in blood group serology

Immune response the body reaction to an antigen; it may be non-specific as in the case of interferon production during viral infections, or specific as in the case of a specific B cell or T cell response

Immune state a biological state in a host who encountered an antigen once and responded to it immunologically; sometimes used to refer to the partial or complete protection against diseases which develops after a prophylactic immunization course

Immunity non-susceptibility to a disease-causing agent

Immunization the production of protection against a pathogen either by active administration of an antigen to a host, or by passive transfer of specific antibody raised against the antigen in another host

Immunocompetence the capacity of a host to produce a normal immune response to an antigen

Immunocompetent cell a cell in the body which can recognize an antigen and mount an immune response to it

Immunodeficiency a deficiency state involving one or more components of the specific of non-specific immune system

Immunoelectrophoresis a technique for separating proteins and other substances in a mixture by electrophoresis and then precipitating them as a precipitin arc pattern by reacting them with antibodies present in an antiserum

Immunofluorescence a technique for visualizing an antigen-antibody reaction by conjugating one of them with a fluorochrome reagent. By using known reagents the test can be adapted for detection of either an antigen or an antibody

Immunogen a substance which can stimulate a specific immune response when introduced into the body

Immunological memory the phenomenon of memory that occurs in a host, following a specific immune response, whereby future contact with the antigen results in a fast and more powerful response; essentially related to the presence of memory small lymphocytes resulting from the previous contact between the immune system and the antigen

Immunological tolerance an immune phenomenon whereby contact between the immune system and an antigen specifically results in loss of capacity of the immune system to react to that particular antigen on subsequent encounter, the immune response to other unrelated antigens being unaffected

Immunoprophylaxis the prevention of disease by use of vaccines or therapeutic antisera

Immunosuppression generalized depression of the immune system by drugs, diseases, poor nutritional state, irradiation etc.

Immunotherapy treatment of disease by specific or non-specific, or active or passive, immunization

Inactivation a procedure which destroys the biological activity of a substance

Inbred strain a line of experimental animals resulting from brother-sister mating for 20 or more generations; such animals are so homogeneous that grafts can be exchanged between them without rejection

Incompatibility antigenic non-identity between two individuals (e.g. donor and recipient of a graft) due to their genetic differences

Incomplete antibody an antibody which cannot link particulate antigens in a saline agglutination test, usually due to certain properties of the antigen against which it has been formed; either there are only a few antigenic determinants on the antigen to promote the reaction, or they are so placed on the antigen surface that there is physical obstruction to the linking of the particles

Indirect Coombs test = indirect type of antiglobulin test *q.v.*

Indirect immunofluorescent antibody technique any fluorescent antibody technique other than the direct or single-layer immunofluorescent technique

Interferon a protein secreted by most healthy cells when infected with a virus

Isoagglutinin isoantibody which can agglutinate isoantigens

Isoantibody any antibody against an isoantigen

Isoantigen an antigen carried by an individual which is capable of eliciting an immune response in individuals of the same species who are genetically different and who do not possess that antigen

Isogeneic = syngeneic *q.v.*

Kinins peptides causing vasodilatation, increased vascular permeability, and smooth muscle contraction; converted from kininogens by certain esterases

Large lymphocyte a lymphocyte with a diameter of 12 μ or more which can be derived by immune stimulation or malignant transformation of either T or B small lymphocytes

Latex agglutination test a test in which a soluble antigen adsorbed onto polystyrene-latex particles is used to detect its specific antibody by agglutination

LE cell a neutrophil leucocyte which has phagocytosed nuclear material combined with IgG antibodies (called antinuclear antibody). The cells occur in many cases of active SLE (systemic lupus erythematosus), but also in some liver diseases, in connective tissue diseases such as rheumatoid arthritis, and in patients on certain drug therapy

Lepromin test a delayed hypersensitivity skin test using an intradermal injection of lepromin, which is an extract of a *M leprae*-containing skin nodule from a patient with lepromatous leprosy

Low-dose tolerance = split tolerance; immunological tolerance induced by exposure of a host to continuous or repeated small doses of an antigen so that future exposure to an optimal immunogenic dose of the same antigen fails to elicit an immune response

Lymphocyte transformation the conversion of a small lymphocyte to a large, primitive-looking blast cell

Lymphokines the products of activated T lymphocytes other than antibodies

Lysosome a membrane-bound cytoplasmic organelle present in many cells, including macrophages, and containing acid hydrolases and other proteases which, in the case of macrophages, are involved in intracellular digestion of phagocytosed material

Lysozyme an enzymic substance (secreted by macrophages) in tears, and nasal and skin secretions, which is bacteriolytic (especially to gram-positive cocci)

Macroglobulin a globulin with a molecular weight above 400 000, e.g. IgM, a_2 macroglobulin, and some serum lipoproteins

Macrophage a mononuclear phagocytic cell of the reticuloendothelial system, derived from the blood monocyte, which is itself a product of the haematopoietic stem cell

Monocyte a large, mononuclear, mobile phagocytic white blood cell, of marrow origin

Multiple myeloma a disease characterized by neoplastic proliferation of plasma cells, which often secrete a homogeneous single type of whole immunoglobulin or discrete components of one

Neutrophil leucocyte a mobile, phagocytic, and short-lived white blood cell of the myeloid series

Nonspecific immunity a body protective mechanism which does not require recognition of a specific organism or antigen

Non-sterilizing immunity = premunition = concomitant immunity *q.v.*

Opsonins substances such as antibody or an activated complement factor which combine with an antigen to facilitate its phagocytosis

Particulate antigen an antigen insoluble in a given fluid medium so that it appears as a suspension rather than a solution; such antigens are usually larger than their colloid equivalents. A soluble antigen can be converted to a particulate state by adsorbing it on to some particulate matter such as latex particles or red cells

Passive immunity immunity transferred from an immune to a non-immune host so that the latter is temporarily immune to the antigen concerned. This process does not involve antigen-specific lymphocytic response or memory and the host responds to future contact with the antigen with a primary immune response

Pathogenicity the capacity of an organism or its products to cause disease

Peripheral lymphoid organs = secondary lymphoid organs; the organs in which the lymphocytes are immunocompetent and therefore capable of responding to antigenic stimulation

Phagocyte a cell which is able to ingest particulate material

PPD purified protein derivative—see tuberculin

Precipitin an antibody which precipitates an antigen when reacted with it

Premunition = concomitant immunity *q.v.*

Primary immune response an immune response occurring at the first contact with an antigen

Primed animal = sensitized animal; an animal which has previously encountered and reacted to an antigen and therefore carries memory cells for response to such an antigen in future

Primed lymphocyte a memory lymphocyte which will respond promptly to a subsequent antigenic stimulus

Radioimmunoassay a method of measuring antigen or antibody using radiolabelled reagents

Reaginic antibody an antibody which fixes to tissue mast cells and basophils of the same species and is involved in immediate hypersensitivity reactions

Receptor a biochemical grouping on a cell membrane which promotes specific reaction at this site with a particular molecule; the latter may be an antigenic determinant, the Fc region of an immunoglobulin, an activated complement factor, etc.

Recognition site the location of an antigenic receptor on a lymphocyte which allows the recognition of antigens in the host

Secondary immune response second or subsequent response of a previously sensitized or primed host to an antigen

Sedimentation coefficient the rate of settling of a molecule under certain defined centrifuging conditions; dependent on weight, size, and shape of molecule

Self-antigen antigens derived from an individual's own tissues

Self-tolerance = autotolerance *q.v.*

Sensitization exposure of a host to an antigen so as to induce an active immune response with memory

Sensitized cell a cell which has reacted with its specific antibody

Sensitized lymphocyte a lymphocyte which has been antigenically primed

Serotherapy use of a serum or antiserum in prophylaxis or treatment

Sterilizing immunity a protective state against a pathogen which follows vaccination, infection, or disease, without the persistence of the pathogen in the immune host

Super antigen an antigen of which the immunogenicity has been increased

Syngeneic genetically identical, e.g. from prolonged inbreeding, or as in monozygotic twins

T cell T lymphocyte or thymus-derived cell

Thymectomy surgical removal of the thyroid

Thymoma a tumour of the thymus

Tolerance = immunological tolerance

Toxoid a bacterial exotoxin which is detoxicated by special procedures to allow its safe use in immunization against the disease it causes

Transfer factor a soluble substance secreted by, or extracted from, primed T lymphocytes; injected into a non-immune host it induces passive cell-mediated immunity

Transplantation antigen = histocompatibility antigen *q.v.*

Tritiated thymidine thymidine labelled with the radioisotope tritium (H_3); used to detect dividing cells, since it is taken up by dividing DNA as the thymidine base and incorporated in the nuclei of the newly found cells

Tuberculin a protein mixture derived from human *M. tuberculosis* and used to detect sensitivity to it in humans

Tuberculin test a skin test using tuberculin

Unprimed = unsensitized or non-sensitized; having had no, or insufficient, contact with an antigen to respond to it

Vaccination exposure of a host to certain live, dead, or detoxified agents to induce active immunity to them or their pathogenic counterparts

Vaccine the therapeutic material used for vaccination

Vaccinia a derivative of cowpox used to produce immunity against smallpox by virtue of the many common antigens it shares with virulent smallpox virus

Valency a term applied to antigen or antibody; when applied to a bacterial cell or red cell antigen, e.g. it refers to the number of antigens of a particular kind present; in case of an antibody it refers to the number of antigen-binding sites in a molecule

Vasoactive amines substances such as 5-hydroxytryptamine (5HT) and histamine, which cause vasodilatation and increased vascular permeability

Warm antibodies antibodies which react at 37°C

Xenograft = heterograft; tissue for grafting between organisms of different species

Zymosan a polysaccharide from yeast cell walls

Self-assessment

Mark the correct answers (more than one may be correct).

1. *The following generally respond to an antigenic stimulus in vivo*
    (a) Brain
    (b) Plasma cells
    (c) T cells of thymus
    (d) T cells of spleen and lymph nodes
    (e) B cells of marrow, spleen, lymph nodes, tonsils.

2. *Passive immunity*
    (a) is acquired protection induced by a course of vaccination
    (b) denotes natural immunity of an infant derived from maternal antibodies
    (c) is life-long due to long-lived memory cells
    (d) is short-lived immunity with lack of memory cell formation
    (e) requires recognition of the antigen by the host lymphocytes.

3. *T helper cells are necessary for*
    (a) IgM response to all antigens
    (b) IgG response to all antigens
    (c) development of memory cell response to all antigens
    (d) formation of T suppressor cells necessary for immune regulation
    (e) low-zone tolerance in the state of autotolerance to many substances.

4. *Viral infections induce immunity by*
    (a) inducing antibody response which neutralizes the multi-

plying intracellular virus

(b) inducing interferon secretion which prevents viral synthesis

(c) inducing cell-mediated immunity to deal with the intracellular phase of the infection

(d) causing immunosuppression in T and B cells

(e) stimulating adequate antibody response to control the viraemic phase.

5. *Cell-mediated immunity*

(a) is particularly defensive against diffusing toxins in the body

(b) handles infections caused by intracellular pathogens

(c) can be tested *in vivo* by a skin test which may show a positive reaction within 15–30 minutes

(d) can be tested *in vivo* by a skin test which may show a positive reaction within 24–48 hours

(e) is mediated by activated macrophages which show enhanced phagocytic capacity and increased capacity for intracellular killing.

6. *A teenager with a history of recurrent bacterial infections since childhood, resistant to antibiotic therapy, and enlarged neck glands suggests*

(a) congenital T cell deficiency

(b) a defect of phagocytosis or complement system

(c) a lymphoreticular malignancy in an immunodeficient patient

(d) autoimmune disease

(e) a defect in humoral immunity.

7. *Premunition or concomitant immunity as seen in parasitic infections reflects*

(a) poor, short-lived memory response in the host against the infective stage of the parasite

(b) good, long-lived memory response in the host against the infective stage of the parasite

(c) the necessity for low-grade parasitaemia in the host to maintain immunity against fresh infections

(d) the necessity for some parasites to survive in an immune host to provide a continuous antigenic stimulus

(e) complete sterile immunity as seen in cutaneous leishmaniasis caused by *L tropica*.

8. *A precipitation or agglutination reaction showing presence of antibody in a serum reflects*

(a) the presence of active disease or previous contact with the antigen concerned

(b) absence of active disease or previous infection

(c) active disease if there is rising titre over a short period

(d) a defensive antibody consistently

(e) any class of antibody which have more than 2 antigen-binding fragments.

Match columns A and B.

9.   A
( ) 1. Fc region
( ) 2. Lysosomes
( ) 3. Fab region
( ) 4. Hinge region

                    B
(a) of IgM antibodies is the site for complement system activation

(b) provides flexibility of an antibody molecule for reaction with an antigen

(c) occurs only in secretory IgA

(d) is the site for antigen-binding in antigen-antibody reaction

(e) are the proteolytic substances of macrophages.

10.

A	B
( ) 1. Alternative pathway of complement	(a) does not require an antigen-antibody reaction for activation
( ) 2. Secondary immune response	(b) is activated by all antigen-antibody responses
( ) 3. Interferon	(c) is only activated by immune complexes with IgG and IgM antibodies
( ) 4. Classical pathway of complement	(d) is also one of the lymphokines
	(e) occurs rapidly, acquiring high levels of long-lasting antibody response.

11.

A	B
( ) 1. Antigenic receptors of B cells	(a) Fc region of IgE
( ) 2. Cell membrane receptors on phagocytes for opsonization	(b) 7S IgM subunits
	(c) Fc region of IgG and C_{3b}
( ) 3. Cell membrane receptors on mast cells and basophils	(d) reflects B cell memory responses
( ) 4. Germinal centres of lymphoid follicles	(e) ankylosing spondylitis.

12.   A   B
( ) 1. Polymorphonuclear   (a) occur at site of immune-
       cells   complex deposits in tissues
( ) 2. Mast cells   (b) supply the J chain of sec-
( ) 3. Eosinophils   retory IgA
( ) 4. Epithelial mucosal   (c) supply the secretory piece
       cells   of secretory IgA
                                      (d) have membrane receptors
                                          for IgE antibodies
                                      (e) can neutralize vasoactive
                                          amines released by mast
                                          cells.

13.   A   B
( ) 1. Immunological sur-   (a) eradicates foci of neo-
       veillance   plastic cells as they arise
( ) 2. Immunological toler-   (b) generalized depression of
       ance   immune system
( ) 3. Immunological sup-   (c) is antigen-specific non-res-
       pression   ponsiveness of the immune
( ) 4. Clonal selection   system
                                      (d) one lymphocyte in 10^4 –
                                          10^5 can respond to an
                                          antigen
                                      (e) is mediated by a lympho-
                                          kine.

14.   A   B
( ) 1. Live attenuated vac-   (a) *Bordetella pertussis* vac-
        cines   cine
( ) 2. Detoxified toxins   (b) vaccine for diphtheria and
( ) 3. Killed organisms   tetanus
( ) 4. Serum sickness   (c) a complication of repeated
                                           use of heterologous ATS
                                      (d) smallpox, yellow fever,
                                           measles, BCG
                                      (e) one dose is often sufficient
                                           for effective vaccination.

15.   A   B
( ) 1. Rheumatoid factor   (a) myasthenia gravis without
( ) 2. Mitochondrial antibody   thymoma
( ) 3. Anti-striated muscle   (b) myasthenia gravis with
        antibody   thymoma
( ) 4. Anti-I antibody   (c) excludes gall stones in a
                                           case of obstructive jaundice
                                      (d) is anti-IgG antibody
                                      (e) a cold antibody.

Answers

1. d, e (pp 1.10 and 1.11).
2. b, d (pp 1.5 and 1.15).
3. b, c, e (pp 2.23, 2.23 and 8.5 resp).
4. b, c, e (pp 4.4, 3.11 and 3.12).
5. b, d, e (pp 3.3, 3.2, 3.9).
6. b, c (p 10.10, Table 10.3, and p 10.14).
7. a, c (p 5.3).
8. a, c, e (pp A.2–A.4).
9. a, e, d, b (p 2.17, Table 10.2, p 2.6, and p 2.3).
10. a, e, d, c (pp 2.28, 1.17, Table 3.1, and p 2.28).
11. b, c, a, d (p 2.26, Table 3.3, Fig 7.1, and p 2.23).
12. a, d, e, c (Table 7.1, Fig 7.1, pp 7.7, 2.14, 3.4 and 6.2).
13. a, c, b, d (pp 3.4, 6.2, 8.1, 8.1 and 1.13).
14. d and e, b, a, c (pp 4.12 and 4.11, Table 4.1. Table 4.1, p 7.16).
15. d, c, b, e (Table 9.3 for d, c, b and e, p 9.7).

Index